SAFETY AND RISK IN SOCIETY

ADULTS GONE MISSING: ALERT SYSTEMS AND FEDERAL ASSISTANCE

SAFETY AND RISK IN SOCIETY

Additional books in this series can be found on Nova's website under the Series tab.

Additional E-books in this series can be found on Nova's website under the E-books tab.

LAWS AND LEGISLATION

Additional books in this series can be found on Nova's website under the Series tab.

Additional E-books in this series can be found on Nova's website under the E-books tab.

SAFETY AND RISK IN SOCIETY

ADULTS GONE MISSING: ALERT SYSTEMS AND FEDERAL ASSISTANCE

THOMAS S. CABRERA
EDITOR

Nova Science Publishers, Inc.
New York

For permission to use material from this book please contact us:
Telephone 631-231-7269; Fax 631-231-8175
Web Site: http://www.novapublishers.com

Additional color graphics may be available in the e-book version of this book.

Library of Congress Cataloging-in-Publication Data

Adults gone missing : alert systems and federal assistance / editor, Thomas S. Cabrera.
p. cm.
Includes index.
ISBN 978-1-62100-085-3 (softcover)
1. Missing persons--United States. 2. Missing persons--Investigation--United States. 3. Alzheimer's disease--Patients--United States. 4. Older people--United States. 5. Emergency communication systems--United States. 6. Emergency management--United States. I. Cabrera, Thomas S.
HV6762.U5A28 2011
363.2'3360973--dc23
2011030088

Published by Nova Science Publishers, Inc. † New York

CONTENTS

PREFACE

A patchwork of alert systems to recover vulnerable missing adults is developing through the country. These systems, administered at the state and local levels, are intended to alert law enforcement entities and the public that adults with cognitive impairment or other disabilities are missing and may need assistance. The alerts are activated on behalf of targeted groups of individuals, such as those with cognitive or mental impairment, developmental disabilities, or suicidal tendencies, who may be at high risk of going missing and unable to make their way home or to a safe place. This book provides an overview of the alert systems, including the legal authority to establish the systems; the target population for the alerts; administrative responsibility for the alerts including coordination with AMBER alerts; training of law enforcement agencies and other entities about the alerts; the process of activating the alerts and coordination of alerts with other states.

Chapter 1- A patchwork of alert systems to recover vulnerable missing adults is developing through the country. These systems, administered at the state and local levels, are intended to alert law enforcement entities and the public that adults with cognitive impairment or other disabilities are missing and may need assistance. The alerts are activated on behalf of targeted groups of individuals—such as those with cognitive or mental impairment (e.g., Alzheimer's disease and other forms of dementia), developmental disabilities, or suicidal tendencies—who may be at high risk of going missing and unable to make their way home or to a safe place.

Chapter 2- Adults may go missing due to choice, an abduction, foul play, a mental or physical disability, or a natural catastrophe, among other reasons. Although no accurate estimates exist of the number of missing adults, the Federal Bureau of Investigation (FBI) reported that as of January 1, 2011, nearly 50,000 missing adult cases were pending in the National Crime

Information Center (NCIC) system, a federal computerized index with data on crimes and locator files for missing and unidentified persons. Certain adults are particularly vulnerable to missing episodes; for example, those with dementia are at risk for wandering. Adults who engage in high-risk behaviors, including involvement in gang activity, may also be more prone to going missing.

In: Adults Gone Missing
Editor: Thomas S. Cabrera

ISBN: 978-1-62100-085-3

Chapter 1

ALERT SYSTEMS FOR MISSING ADULTS IN ELEVEN STATES: BACKGROUND AND ISSUES FOR CONGRESS*

Adrienne L. Fernandes and Kirsten J. Colello

SUMMARY

A patchwork of alert systems to recover vulnerable missing adults is developing through the country. These systems, administered at the state and local levels, are intended to alert law enforcement entities and the public that adults with cognitive impairment or other disabilities are missing and may need assistance. The alerts are activated on behalf of targeted groups of individuals—such as those with cognitive or mental impairment (e.g., Alzheimer's disease and other forms of dementia), developmental disabilities, or suicidal tendencies—who may be at high risk of going missing and unable to make their way home or to a safe place.

Recent media attention to cases of vulnerable missing adults has prompted policymakers to consider whether the federal government should expand its role in helping these individuals. Currently, the federal Missing Alzheimer's Disease Patient Alert program funds a service that provides enrollees—

---

* This is an edited, reformatted and augmented version of a Congressional Research Service publication, report R40552, dated May 7, 2011.

individuals with Alzheimer's or dementia—with a bracelet indicating that the individual is memory impaired, including a toll-free, 24-hour emergency response number to call if the person is found wandering or lost.

Some Members of Congress have expressed interest in assisting states to create and expand alert systems for missing adults. In the opening weeks of the 111th Congress, the House passed legislation (H.R. 632) to establish a grant program to encourage states to develop, expand, and coordinate these alert systems. A companion bill (S. 557) was introduced in the Senate shortly thereafter. The proposed program is similar to a federal grant program that funds training and technical assistance for what are known as AMBER (America's Missing: Broadcast Emergency Response) Alert systems. Each state has developed an AMBER Alert system to assist in the recovery of children who are believed to have been abducted.

In response to the increased congressional focus on alert systems for missing adults, the Congressional Research Service (CRS) gathered data on 11 states (Colorado, Delaware, Florida, Georgia, Kentucky, North Carolina, Ohio, Oklahoma, Rhode Island, Texas, and Virginia) that were known to have developed such systems. CRS conducted a review of state laws, regulations, or executive orders that established the systems, and contacted officials in each of the states to learn more about how the systems were administered. CRS found that most of the systems were established only recently, since 2006.

This report provides an overview of the alert systems in these 11 states, including (1) the legal authority to establish the systems; (2) the target population for the alerts; (3) administrative responsibility for the alerts, including coordination with AMBER Alerts; (4) training of law enforcement agencies and other entities about the alerts; (5) the process for activating alerts; (6) coordination of alerts with other states; (7) system costs; (8) use of the systems; and (9) any information about outcomes of the individuals for whom alerts were activated.

The last section of the report provides a discussion of issues for Congress to consider with respect to the federal role, if any, in developing state alert programs for missing adults. For example, some states with alert systems noted that they might have difficulty coordinating with another state that lacks a similar system. States may also have challenges coordinating with states that have alert systems with different criteria that must be met before an alert is activated. The federal government may be able to help establish protocols to coordinate cross-state alerts and to assist in establishing formal agreements or protocols for the use of interstate alerts.

INTRODUCTION

Adults may go missing for a variety of reasons. In some cases, the disappearance of an individual may be a personal choice. However, adults may go missing as a result of a disabling condition, a natural catastrophe, or a crime such as an abduction and other instances when foul play is involved. Unlike children, adults have the legal right to go missing under most circumstances. As a result, families of missing adults may receive limited assistance from state and local law enforcement agencies in recovering their loved ones.

Media attention to cases of missing adults—particularly seniors with dementia who have been found deceased after wandering from home either on foot or in a vehicle—has prompted policymakers to consider expanding the federal government's role in helping to recover vulnerable adults who go missing. Congress has recently proposed measures to assist in such recovery efforts. At the start of the 111th Congress, the House passed legislation (H.R. 632) to establish a grant program to encourage states to establish, expand, and coordinate alert systems for vulnerable adults who may go missing due to cognitive or physical disabilities, among other reasons.[1] A companion bill (S. 557) was introduced in the Senate on March 10, 2009. The proposed program is similar to a federal grant program that funds training and technical assistance for what are known as AMBER (America's Missing: Broadcast Emergency Response) Alert systems. Each state has developed an AMBER Alert system to enlist the support of law enforcement agencies and the public in recovering children who are believed to have been abducted.

In response to the increased congressional focus on alert systems for missing adults, the Congressional Research Service (CRS) gathered data on existing state alert systems in 11 states. CRS conducted a review of state laws, regulations, or executive orders that established the systems, and contacted officials in the 11 states to learn more about how they are carried out. These systems were established beginning in 2006, and are administered by local and/or state law enforcement agencies. The systems are intended to alert law enforcement entities and/or the public that vulnerable adults are missing and may need assistance. Many states activate the alerts on behalf of targeted groups of individuals who may be at high risk of going missing, such as those persons with cognitive or mental impairment, including Alzheimer's and other forms of dementia, as well as persons with developmental disability.

This report provides an overview of the alert systems in 11 states. It begins with background information on current federal efforts to recover missing adults, followed by a description of the methods CRS used to obtain data from each state identified as having an alert system. Subsequent sections of this report provide an overview of each state's alert systems, including (1) the legal authority to establish the systems; (2) the target population for the alerts; (3) administrative responsibility for the alerts, including coordination with AMBER Alerts; (4) training of law enforcement agencies and other entities about the alerts; (5) the process for activating alerts; (6) coordination of alerts with other states; (7) system costs; (8) use of the systems; and (9) any information about outcomes of the individuals who were believed to be lost and for whom alerts were activated. The last section of the report provides a discussion of issues for Congress to consider with respect to the federal role, if any, in developing state alert systems for missing adults.

Background

Individuals can go missing for a variety of reasons. They may become lost or disoriented due to a mental or cognitive impairment, developmental disability, or physical disability. Natural disasters, such as hurricanes or floods, may cause individuals to become displaced from their families and communities. Individuals may voluntarily go missing to escape domestic abuse, law enforcement, or for other reasons. Policymakers and advocates for the missing have identified persons with Alzheimer's disease and other forms of dementia as being particularly vulnerable to missing episodes.[2] Increases in longevity among the older population and the aging of the baby boom generation have contributed to interest in establishing these systems. Wandering from home can be a frequent behavior that may pose a significant, sometimes life-threatening, danger to the wellbeing of those with Alzheimer's disease and other forms of dementia. According to the Alzheimer's Association, if not found within 24 hours, nearly 50% of those who wander risk serious illness or death.[3] Illness or death may occur from exposure to the elements, lack of food or hydration for an extended period, and general inability of the individual to think, act, or communicate to gain assistance.

While local and state law enforcement agencies are responsible for leading efforts to recover missing adults, in recent years the federal government has increasingly played a role in both helping to prevent certain types of missing adult incidents—particularly among vulnerable populations—and assisting in identifying and recovering those who go missing.[4] The federal Missing Alzheimer's Disease Patient Alert grant assists in identifying missing individuals with Alzheimer's disease and other forms of dementia by funding what is known as Safe Return, a program administered by the Alzheimer's Association. Safe Return provides a MedicAlert bracelet or other form of identification to enrolled individuals. The identification indicates that the individual is memory impaired and includes a toll-free, 24-hour emergency response number to call if the person is found wandering or lost. As part of the program, the Alzheimer's Association provides support and referrals to caregivers of those enrolled in the program, and provides some training to law enforcement agencies about individuals with Alzheimer's disease. Authorization for the program has lapsed, but Congress has continued to appropriate funds. For each of FY2002 through FY2009 Congress appropriated between $800,000 and $2 million in funding. The Missing Alzheimer's Disease Patient Alert Program Reauthorization of 2009 (H.R. 908), which was approved by the House on February 10, 2009, would amend the Violent Crime Control and Law Enforcement Act of 1994 to reauthorize the program through FY2016, and would revise program requirements to: (1) provide for competitive grants to nonprofit organizations to assist in locating missing patients with Alzheimer's disease and related dementia; (2) expand the program to include locating other missing elderly individuals; and (3) establish a preference in awarding grants to national nonprofit organizations that have a direct link to patients with Alzheimer's disease and related dementias and their families. Currently, grants may be awarded to only such organizations.

Separately, Congress provided funding from FY2002 through FY2006 for the Kristen's Act grant program which provided funding for a national clearinghouse and resource center for missing adults generally. Federal funding for Kristen's Act grants ranged from a high of $1.7 million in FY2002, decreasing in each subsequent year to a low of $150,000 in FY2006. The National Center for Missing Adults (NCMA) was the sole recipient of the grant. NCMA continues to operate, with non-federal funds, and takes reports of persons who go missing under a variety of circumstances, including due to a diagnosed medical condition, mental illness or diminished mental capacity, Alzheimer's disease or dementia, or alcohol or substance abuse.[5] NCMA adds profiles and pictures of missing persons to its website (http://www.missing adults.org), sends missing person flyers to the family and law enforcement, assists with press releases, helps generate or manage media attention, and maintains routine contact with the families of missing individuals. Authorization for Kristen's Act expired in FY2006. H.R. 632, which passed the House on February 10, 2009, would reauthorize the grant at $4 million for each of FY2010 through FY2020. Companion legislation, S. 557, was introduced in the Senate on March 10, 2008.

In addition to funding the Kristen's Act grant, H.R. 632 would direct the Attorney General to establish a national "Silver Alert communications network" to assist regional and local search efforts for missing seniors, in coordination with states, local governments, and law enforcement agencies. The bill defines "missing senior" as any individual who is reported to, or identified by, a law enforcement agency as a missing person; and meets the requirements to be designated as a missing senior, as determined by the state in which the individual is reported or identified as a missing person. The bill further directs the Department of Justice (DOJ) to appoint a National Coordinator of the network to: (1) establish voluntary guidelines for states to use in developing alert programs to recover missing seniors; (2) develop protocols for recovering missing seniors and for notifying law enforcement agencies that a senior is missing; and (3) implement an advisory group to assist states, local governments, law enforcement agencies, and other entities involved in the network, among other activities. The bill authorizes such sums as necessary for these purposes. No time period is specified. In addition, H.R. 632 would authorize appropriations of $5 million annually for FY2009 through FY2013 for grants to states to develop and enhance Silver Alert plans. The grants would be distributed by DOJ on an equitable basis throughout the United States. The federal share of the grant would not exceed 50%.

The focus of this report is on those state alert systems for missing adults. CRS sought to obtain detailed information from states about their alert systems to better inform Congress about their activities as well as analyze the similarities and differences among various state alert systems. In general, these alert systems are intended to rapidly disperse information about a missing person to law enforcement entities, and often the public. This type of alert system is different from the federally funded Safe Return program in that Safe Return maintains a database of individuals who have been pre-identified as being at risk of wandering due to Alzheimer's disease and related dementia and choose to enroll in the program. In the event that an individual enrolled in the Safe Return program does go missing, Safe Return can provide information and a physical description of the missing individual, which can assist family members in filing a missing persons report and help law enforcement agencies, regardless of whether the state has an alert system, in search and recovery efforts. Provided that the missing individual is wearing identification, Safe Return can also facilitate reuniting missing persons with their caregivers.

METHODOLOGY

Based on requests from some Members of Congress for information regarding the administration of alert systems for missing adults, CRS sought to identify states that were believed to have missing adult alert systems and contact those states to obtain further information. Using information from a variety of sources, including recent news articles, policy publications, and discussions with various stakeholders from organizations such as the Alzheimer's Association and Project Lifesaver International, Inc.,[6] CRS identified 11 states with alert systems for missing adults—Colorado, Delaware, Florida, Georgia, Kentucky, North Carolina, Ohio, Oklahoma, Rhode Island, Texas, and Virginia.[7] CRS did not conduct a search of state statutes or survey all 50 states to determine whether each state had implemented an alert system for missing adults. Thus, the 11 identified states may not be an exhaustive list of all states with alert systems for vulnerable missing adults.

For the 11 selected states, CRS reviewed authorizing legislation, executive orders, and regulations to obtain program data on these state alert systems. CRS also contacted officials in each of the states to obtain additional information. Based on key areas of interest in state alert systems for missing adults that have been expressed by some Members of Congress, CRS prepared a detailed list of questions for state officials covering the following attributes (see Appendix A for a copy of the questions submitted to state officials):

1. Legal authority—whether authority for implementation and administration of the alert system was established by the state through statute, executive order, and/or regulations.
2. Target population—information on the characteristics of those who may go missing and the population eligible to be the subject of an alert.
3. Administrative responsibility—the entity or entities responsible for implementation of and administering the alert system and any administrative coordination with the state's AMBER Alert program.
4. Training—any training provided to law enforcement agencies and other stakeholders on the use of the alert system.
5. Process for activating alerts—includes information on: eligible entities authorized to file an actionable missing persons report; criteria for activating an alert; communication mechanisms for disseminating the alert; target audiences; and duration of the alert.

6. Interstate coordination—any state protocols for alert systems to coordinate with other states when an eligible missing person is believed to have crossed state lines.
7. System costs—costs associated with implementing the alert system as well as any costs for ongoing administration of the system.
8. Use of the system—the history of utilization of the alert system including any available data on the number of alerts that have been activated.
9. Outcomes—any available data on: the characteristics of those missing individuals who are the subject of an alert; circumstances related to their disappearance; and outcomes related to any search and recovery efforts.

Between September 2008 and March 2009, questions were electronically submitted to the state official identified by CRS as responsible for or most knowledgeable about the missing adult alert system in that state. All 11 states responded and, when necessary, CRS followed up with state officials for clarification. Officials provided varying levels of detail about their systems. For some states, CRS was unable to obtain information about the number of alerts activated and/or the costs associated with the alert system.

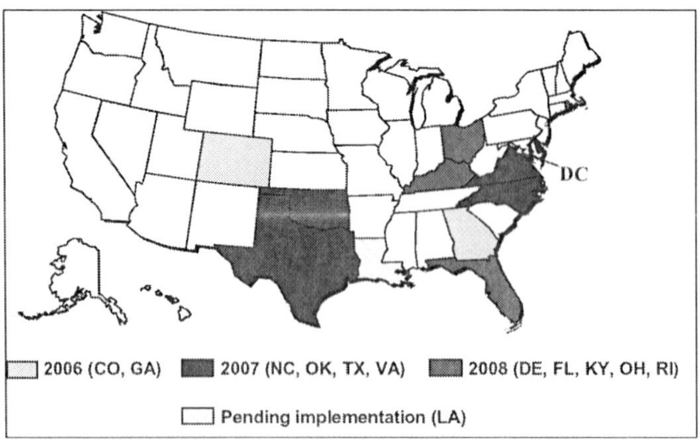

Source: Congressional Research Service based on correspondence with state officials from September 2008 through March 2009.

Notes: States identified as having an alert system for missing adults represent a convenience sample.

Figure 1. Geographic Distribution of States with Alert Systems for Missing Adults (by year of implementation).

Overview of State Alert Systems

Alert systems for vulnerable missing adults appear to be a recent but growing initiative. Among the 11 states CRS identified with active alert systems, Colorado and Georgia were the first to implement an alert system for missing vulnerable adults in 2006. Since then, nine other states have adopted the systems. Eight of the 11 states are in the South (Delaware, Florida, Georgia, Kentucky, North Carolina, Oklahoma, Texas, and Virginia), one state is in the West (Colorado), one state is in the Midwest (Ohio), and one state is in the Northeast (Rhode Island).[8] See **Figure 1** for a U.S. map with the 11 states identified by CRS as having missing adult alert systems.

Table 1 provides a general overview of the alert systems implemented in the 11 states identified by CRS as having active programs. State alert systems were authorized either by law or executive order, with most states passing a law to create the alert system for missing adults.

Table 1. Summary of Selected States' Alert Systems for Missing Adults

State	Description of Alert System
Colorado	In 2006, the state established the Missing Senior Citizen Alert Program, which requires the Colorado Bureau of Investigation (CBI) to disseminate information to alert local law enforcement agencies and the public through the media about certain missing senior citizens. The alert system targets senior citizens with a verified impaired mental condition. The CBI activates the alert at the request of the local law enforcement agency.
Delaware	In 2008, the state established the Delaware Gold Alert Program, which requires local law enforcement agencies to activate a Gold Alert in certain missing person investigation cases. The Gold Alert may be used to assist in locating a missing person with a disability, a missing senior citizen, or missing suicidal person. The investigative law enforcement agency activates the alert in cooperation with the Delaware State Police.
Florida	In 2008, the state established the Florida Silver Alert Plan, which authorizes the state to post information on road signs to alert the public about certain missing persons. The information is posted at the request of local law enforcement agencies in circumstances where a person age 60 or older with

Table 1. (Continued)

State	Description of Alert System
	dementia is missing and under extraordinary circumstances for a missing adult age 15 to 59 with a similar condition. Local law enforcement agencies are encouraged to develop policies and procedures to broadcast information to the public about the missing person in their jurisdictions.
Georgia	In 2006, the state established Mattie's Call, a missing person alert system administered by the Georgia Bureau of Investigation (GBI). Mattie's Call may be used to assist in locating a disabled adult, of any age, who is developmentally impaired or suffers from a cognitive impairment, such as dementia. The alert is activated by the GBI, at the request of a local law enforcement agency, to other law enforcement agencies and the public through media outlets and electronic highway signs.
Kentucky	In 2008, the state established the Golden Alert system. The law requires rescue squads organized to search for a missing impaired adult to cooperate with local media outlets and law enforcement entities. The Golden Alert system targets missing "impaired adults" who are persons age 18 years or older that have a verified mental or cognitive impairment. Local law enforcement agencies determine if a missing person qualifies for an alert and, are responsible for activating the alerts and contacting the media.
North Carolina	In 2007, the state established a Silver Alert Program that activates a missing person alert to appropriate law enforcement agencies, the media, the public, and other entities. The Silver Alert Program targets missing persons, of any age, who are believed to be suffering from dementia or other cognitive impairment. The North Carolina Center for Missing Persons activates the Silver Alert at the request of the investigating law enforcement agency.
Ohio	In 2008, the state established the Ohio Missing Adult Alert system administered by the Bureau of Criminal Identification and Investigation within the office of the Ohio Attorney General. The alert system targets missing individuals age 65 or older, or adults age 18 or older with a mental impairment. Alerts are authorized by a local law enforcement agency and are activated by the Ohio Attorney General's office or the Ohio State Highway Patrol.

State	Description of Alert System
Oklahoma	In 2007, the state established the Silver Alert System. The alert system targets individuals, of any age, with a proven mental or physical disability. At their discretion, the local law enforcement agency activates the alert to other law enforcement agencies and to the public through the media.
Rhode Island	In 2008, the state created the Rhode Island Missing Senior Citizen Alert system administered by the Rhode Island State Police, in coordination with local law enforcement agencies. The target population is seniors age 60 or older who have an impaired mental condition. Upon the request of the state police, the alert is activated to the Rhode Island Broadcasters Association, which in turn disseminates the information to member media outlets. Electronic highway signs may be activated on a case-by-case basis.
Texas	In 2007, the state established the Texas Silver Alert Network administered by the Governor's Division of Emergency Management. The target population are senior citizens, age 65 or older, who are domiciled in Texas, and have a diagnosed impaired mental condition. The alert is activated at the request of a local law enforcement agency, to other law enforcement agencies and the public through the media.
Virginia	In 2007, the state established the Virginia Senior Alert system administered by the Virginia Missing Person Information Clearinghouse within the Virginia Police Department. The Senior Alert system is targeted at missing persons age 60 years or older who suffer a cognitive impairment. The alert is activated by local law enforcement agencies, at their discretion, to other law enforcement agencies and the public through the media. Regional and statewide alerts are activated by the Virginia State Police.

Source: Congressional Research Service based on correspondence with state officials between September 2008 and March 2009.

Notes: For details about specific state alert systems, see **Appendix B.** States identified as having an alert system for missing adults represent a convenience sample.

The administration of state alert systems for missing vulnerable adults appears to be a cooperative effort among state and local law enforcement agencies. These alert systems are intended to rapidly disseminate information to other law enforcement agencies and the public through various media outlets (e.g., television, radio, print media, lottery terminals, electronic highway signs, trucker alert systems) about a missing person by providing descriptive information about the missing person or vehicle, in the event a missing person is believed to be driving. For some states, the impetus for legislation to establish the alert system came as a result of public attention surrounding missing person investigations that involved adults with mental or cognitive impairment.

Multiple states reported that they modeled their missing adult alert systems after their state AMBER Alert systems for abducted children. States indicated that while their alert systems for missing adults are similar to their AMBER Alert systems, AMBER alerts were more widely disseminated. Generally, the same state-level agencies administer or are involved in administering both alert systems, and in some cases, the two systems share one budget. Most states reported that training on the use of the alert system for missing adults is provided to state and/or local law enforcement agencies with some states providing education to the public and other stakeholders.

States have defined their target population for their alert systems differently. Some states include age as a factor for activating an alert, such as the population age 65 and older. Other factors include whether the individual has a cognitive, physical, or developmental disability, or a severe mental health impairment. In general, the process for activating an alert begins with the local law enforcement agency taking a missing persons report (see **Figure 2**). In order for an alert to then be activated, entities at the local and state level, depending on the state's protocol, must ensure that the criteria for activating an alert have been met. States may require that certain individuals file a missing persons report in order to activate the alert system. In most states, verification that the individual has a mental or cognitive impairment can be through a family member, caregiver, or guardian.

One difference among states with alert systems is the designated entity responsible for activating the alert. In six states, a lead state agency is responsible for activating alerts at the request of a local law enforcement agency. The remaining five states have localized models for the dissemination of alerts where the local law enforcement agency activates the alerts locally and/or regionally and may seek assistance from the state law enforcement agency to disseminate the alert statewide. In general, the entity responsible for activating an alert will disseminate the missing person's information to other law enforcement agencies and various media outlets to alert the public. When the public is alerted about the missing information, generally information is publicized on how to contact law enforcement with tips or information.

Most states have some mechanisms in place for coordinating alerts with other states to recover individuals who were believed to have crossed state lines during their disappearance.

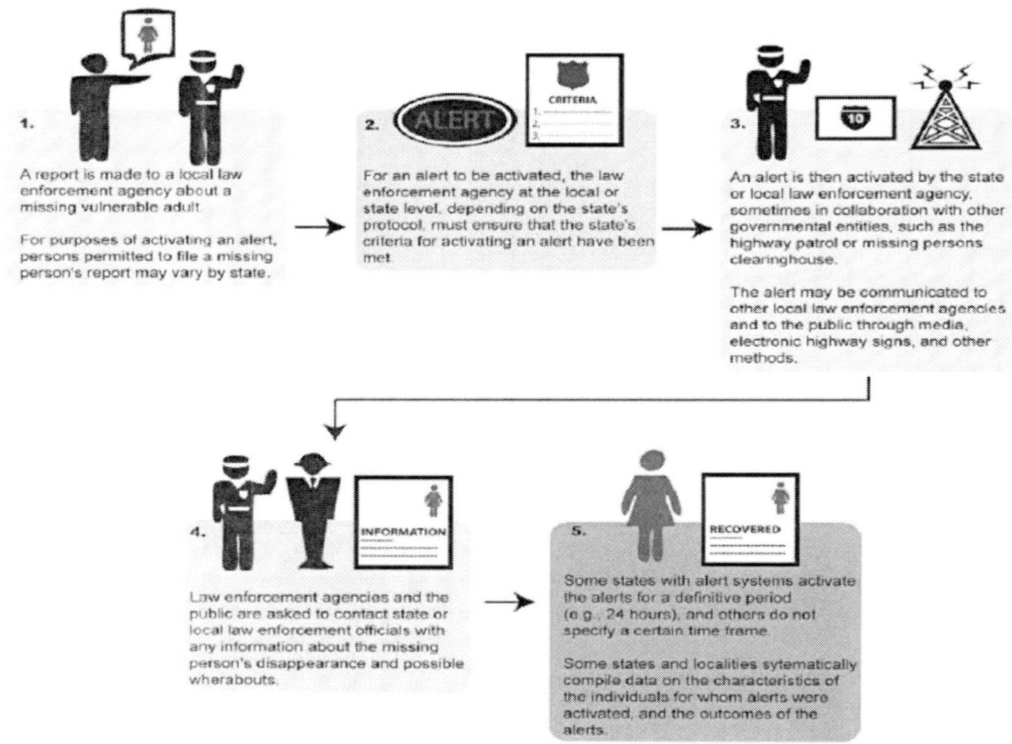

Source: Congressional Research Service.

Note: This diagram is a general depiction of the process for activating an alert, and does not represent the exact process in each state.

Figure 2. Process for Issuing an Alert for Missing Vulnerable Adults.

Several states indicated there was no additional cost to implement the alert system or that implementation costs were absorbed by the existing budget for the AMBER alert program or another program. Some states provided data on the actual costs of operating the alert system. Data from these states estimated that the annual cost of operating an alert system was between $40,000 and $182,000. However, these estimates exclude costs to local law enforcement agencies or other stakeholders that may be involved in helping to administer the alert system.

Ten out of 11 states reported having used the alert system, the exception being Delaware. Although some states reported no information about the number of alerts that have been activated, states that did report this information reported activating anywhere between one (Rhode Island) and 82 alerts (North Carolina) since implementation of their alert system. However, the number of alerts a state has activated is likely affected by how long the system has been active, the process and criteria for activating the alerts, the state's identified target population for the alert, and whether the system is generally accepted by law enforcement agencies and other stakeholders as a viable tool to assist in the recovery of missing vulnerable adults. Most states were able to provide information about the outcomes of recovery efforts for these missing persons with the majority of states reporting that individuals were found recovered, though almost every state reported at least one individual who was found deceased.

Details of State Programs

States provided varying levels of detail about their alert systems. This section summarizes information provided by state officials, including (1) legal authority; (2) target population; (3) administrative responsibility; (4) training; (5) process for activating alerts; (6) interstate coordination; (7) system costs; (8) use of the system; and (9) outcomes. These attributes are described in tables for each state in **Appendix B**.

Legal Authority

Missing adult alert systems appear to be recent initiatives. Among the 11 states CRS identified, two states implemented their alert systems for missing adults in 2006, four states implemented alert systems in 2007, and five states implemented them in 2008. States that adopted these alert systems may have been more likely to be located near states that also have an alert system. In fact, Virginia state officials indicated that their alert system was developed as a result of similar efforts underway in other states. The majority of states with alert systems for missing adults derived their authority to establish the program from enacted law, with two exceptions. In 2006, Oklahoma created a Silver Alert program through a non-binding resolution adopted by the state House of Representatives. In 2008, Florida's governor signed an executive order to establish the state's Silver Alert Plan.

In some cases, the impetus for legislation to establish the alert system came as a result of public attention surrounding missing person investigations that involved adults with mental or cognitive impairment. For example, Georgia's system was established in 2006 in response to a patient with Alzheimer's disease who went missing from her home in 2004. Ohio indicated that their system was developed in response to several incidents throughout the country, as well as elsewhere in Ohio, that involved missing older individuals or individuals with mental impairment. Other states indicated that the need to focus on the senior population as well as advocacy efforts on behalf of seniors was an important consideration for implementation of an alert system. Florida's executive order states that the senior population is growing and that the state needed to implement a standardized system to aid in the search of seniors who go missing. Colorado's authorizing law (S.B. 06-057) states that the program will aid in the recovery of missing seniors within the first few hours of their disappearance, a critical time frame for those with cognitive impairment.

Target Population

In general, state alert systems for missing adults are targeted at a vulnerable population of adults due to advanced age, cognitive, physical, or developmental disability, or a combination of age and disability. However, states have defined their target populations differently. **Table 2** describes the target populations for state alert systems based on age and disability status. Four states (Colorado, Rhode Island, Texas, and Virginia) have alert systems that exclusively target older adults, defined as either 60 or 65 years of age or older with an "impaired mental condition" or "cognitive impairment." Florida and Ohio target older adults, but also provide conditions for activating alerts on behalf of missing younger adults. The remaining five states (Delaware,

Georgia, Kentucky, North Carolina, Oklahoma) have alert systems that can be activated on behalf of adults of any age.

Table 2. Target Population for State's Missing Adult Alert System

State	Age	Disability Status
Colorado	60+	Verified impaired mental condition
Delaware[a]	18+	Disabled
	60+	None Specified
Florida[b]	18 to 59	Irreversible deterioration of mental faculties
	60+	
Georgia	18+	Developmental disability or cognitive impairment
Kentucky	18+	Verified mental or cognitive impairment
North Carolina	18+	Dementia or other cognitive impairment
Ohio	18 to 64	Mental impairment
	65+	None specified
Oklahoma[c]	18+	Mental or physical disability
Rhode Island	60+	Impaired mental condition
Texas	65+	Diagnosed impaired mental condition
Virginia	60+	Cognitive impairment

Source: Congressional Research Service based on correspondence with state officials between September 2008 and March 2009.

a. Delaware's alert system targets three categorical groups: (1) missing senior citizens defined as persons age 60 or older; (2) missing persons with a disability; (3) and missing suicidal persons who are described as persons whose statements, actions, or conduct indicate that the person may voluntarily cause or inflict self-harm.

b. Florida's alert system targets the senior population age 60 or older; however, under extraordinary circumstances an alert can be activated for a missing person age 18 to 59 with irreversible deterioration of mental faculties.

c. Although Oklahoma reported that there are no age criteria for activating an alert, state officials indicated their alert system is primarily targeted at missing elderly.

In all states, alert systems for missing adults are activated on behalf of adults who are disabled due to a mental or cognitive impairment. At least three states activate alerts on behalf of persons with physical disabilities or with severe mental health conditions. Oklahoma activates alerts on behalf of adults with physical disabilities. Georgia will activate an alert for an adult with a developmental disability. And in addition to targeting missing seniors and persons with a disability, Delaware's alert system targets missing suicidal persons. Three states (Georgia, Ohio, and Virginia) provided language defining cognitive or mental impairment (see **Table 3**).

Table 3. Definitions of Cognitive or Mental Impairment in Selected States

State	Definition of Cognitive or Mental Impairment
Georgia	Cognitive impairment refers to diminished conscious intellectual activity (i.e., thinking, reasoning, or remembering).
Ohio	Mental impairment is defined as a substantial disorder of thought, mood, perception, orientation, or memory that grossly impairs judgment, behavior, or ability to live independently, or provide self-care as certified by a licensed physician, psychiatrist, or psychologist.
Virginia	Cognitive impairment refers to Alzheimer's disease or other forms of dementia. The individual must suffer from cognitive impairment to the extent that he or she is unable to provide care to himself or herself without assistance from a caregiver.

Source: Congressional Research Service based on correspondence with state officials between September 2008 and March 2009.

Notes: Three of the 11 states provided a definition of cognitive or mental impairment.

Verification of a cognitive impairment or other disability is often included as part of the state's criteria for activating an alert (see discussion of Criteria for Activating Alert below). Six states (Delaware, Florida, Kentucky, North Carolina, Ohio, and Virginia) indicated that the reporting party attests to the missing person's condition and that this information is then verified by the investigating officer (no further information was provided about how the officer verifies the information). Other states (Oklahoma, Rhode Island, and Texas) require further documentation, such as prescription medications or medical records, in order to verify an individual's condition. Texas reported requiring documentation from a medical or mental health provider regarding the missing senior's condition. To verify an impaired mental condition in Colorado, family members must sign a statement stating that the missing person is mentally impaired. In Georgia verification that the individual has a cognitive impairment or other disability can be made through a family member, caregiver, or guardian, with no further verification by local law enforcement or additional documentation required.

Administrative Responsibility

Administration of a state's alert system is often a cooperative effort among state and local law enforcement agencies. Statewide agencies in six states (Colorado, Georgia, North Carolina, Ohio, Rhode Island, and Texas) take the lead in administering the program and activate alerts at the request of a local law enforcement agency. For example, in North Carolina, the Center for Missing Persons within the state's Department of Crime Control and Safety activates alerts.[9] In Texas, the Governor's Division of Emergency Management activates alerts; however, a local law enforcement agency also has the option of issuing an alert locally or regionally, if they are in area that has a regional alert program for missing seniors. Both Ohio and Texas reported having steering committees that provide guidance to the administering state agencies concerning the alert systems. The committees are comprised of local and state law enforcement agencies and other stakeholders.

In four other states (Delaware, Kentucky, Oklahoma, and Virginia), the local law enforcement agency takes the lead in administering the program and activates the alert locally or regionally, but can also seek assistance from the state law enforcement agency to disseminate the alert statewide or coordinate the alert with other states, if necessary (see section on Interstate Coordination below). Similarly, local law enforcement agencies in Virginia will administer and activate alerts locally and can make requests to the Virginia State Police to activate an alert regionally or statewide. In Oklahoma, local law enforcement agencies administer and activate alerts but may seek assistance from the state's Department of Public Safety in order to disseminate an alert to multiple law enforcement agencies throughout the state.

Finally, Florida's system of administration is somewhat different from the other states. The state's Silver Alert Plan is administered by the state Missing Endangered Persons Information Clearinghouse, within the Florida Department of Law Enforcement (FDLE). A Silver Alert is activated when the local law enforcement agency requests assistance from the Florida Department of Law Enforcement for an alert in multiple regions of the state via electronic highway signs. Alerts may be activated by the state only for persons who are believed to be driving and only alert the public through electronic highway signs and the FLDE website. Separately, local law enforcement agencies may activate a Silver Alert locally based on criteria established by the local law enforcement agencies.

AMBER Alert Coordination

The 11 states provided information about coordination between their missing adult alert systems and AMBER Alert systems for abducted children. AMBER Alert systems are voluntary partnerships—between law enforcement agencies, broadcasters, and transportation agencies—to activate messages in a targeted area when a child is abducted and believed to be in grave danger (see **Figure 3**). Generally, states responded that the same state-level agency administers or is involved with both the AMBER alert and missing adult alert systems, and in some cases, the two systems share a budget. For example, Texas indicated that its Silver Alert Network and its AMBER Alert system are administered by the Governor's Division of Emergency Management, but operate as separate programs.[10] Further, multiple states reported that they modeled their alert systems for missing adults after their AMBER Alert systems. States also reported that law enforcement agencies often disseminate the information to the public through various media using the same communication mechanisms.

State officials identified two major distinctions between missing adult alert and AMBER alert systems. First, five of the states (Colorado, Delaware, Florida, Kentucky, and Texas) indicated that AMBER Alerts are more widely disseminated than alerts for missing adults. For example, Texas officials indicated that both the missing adult alerts and AMBER Alerts are distributed via the media and on billboards and lottery machines. However, AMBER Alerts in the state are additionally distributed through venues including the National Center for Missing and Exploited Children's Secondary Notification System, which notifies numerous stakeholders—law enforcement agencies, public service entities, internet and wireless providers, trucking companies, and others—about the missing child alert.[13]

Second, at least seven of the states (Colorado, Georgia, North Carolina, Ohio, Oklahoma, Texas, and Virginia) use emergency alert system (EAS) technology to report AMBER Alerts, and not alerts about missing adults. (Note that the states were not prompted to provide information about the EAS, and the other four states did not.) The EAS sends emergency messages to the public with the cooperation of broadcast radio and television and most cable television stations.[14] The Federal Communication Commission (FCC) is designated by the Federal Emergency Management Administration (FEMA) to manage broadcaster involvement in EAS. The FCC currently provides technical standards and support for EAS, rules for its operation, and enforcement within the broadcasting and cable industries. According to the

FCC, states and localities are not permitted to use the EAS to broadcast an alert about a missing adult.[15]

AMBER (America's Missing: Broadcast Emergency Response) Alert systems are state administered. Each state, the District of Columbia, Puerto Rico, and the U.S. Virgin Islands have implemented these systems statewide. Some states also have developed regional and local AMBER Alert systems. Federal law authorizes, and Congress has appropriated, funding through the Department of Justice (DOJ) to assist local and state law enforcement agencies in developing and carrying out their programs.[11] Each year since FY2003, funding has been appropriated for federal AMBER Alert activities, which is used to provide training and technical assistance to law enforcement officials. The DOJ has also issued guidance that states should reference in activating AMBER Alerts.[12] Many states follow these guidelines, activating an alert only when an abducted child is believed to be in grave danger and enough descriptive information exists about the victim and the abductor for law enforcement to activate an alert. These alerts are sent to the public via television and radio broadcasts and electronic signs, among other methods. The public is asked to be on the lookout for the abducted child and to contact law enforcement officials with any information about the child's whereabouts.

Source: Congressional Research Service.

Figure 3. Federal Support for AMBER Alert Systems.

Training

States provided varying levels of detail about the type of training and education law enforcement agencies and the public received about the state's alert system for missing vulnerable adults. Eight of the 11 states (Colorado, Delaware, Georgia, Ohio, North Carolina, Rhode Island, Texas, and Virginia) reported that training was provided to state and/or local enforcement agencies. In four of these states, training or educational materials were also provided to the public and other stakeholders. For example, the Colorado Bureau of Investigation provided training or educational materials to law enforcement agencies, the public, media, and the state Alzheimer's Association chapter. Virginia State Police provided training to local law enforcement on the activation criteria and the procedures for activating the alert, while the Attorney General's office provided information to the public about the alert system. Florida state officials reported that funding is currently not available for training, but if funds become available, training on procedures for activating the system will be targeted to law enforcement and transportation officials. Finally, Kentucky and Oklahoma state officials reported that they were uncertain whether local law enforcement agencies received training, and did not provide any further information.

Process for Activating an Alert

There is wide variation among states with respect to the process for activating alerts for vulnerable adults in the 11 states. The following describes the process for activating an alert. This process includes information on: (1) filing an actionable missing persons report; (2) criteria for activating an alert; (3) communication mechanisms for disseminating the alert; (4) target audiences; and (5) duration of the alert.

Filing a Missing Persons Report

In general, the process for activating an alert originates with the local law enforcement agency taking a missing persons report. Seven states (Delaware, Georgia, North Carolina, Oklahoma, Rhode Island, Texas, Virginia) specified that certain individuals must file a missing persons report in order to activate the state or local alert system. For example, in Georgia a family member or caretaker must file a missing person's report. North Carolina requires a parent, spouse, legal guardian or custodian, or person responsible for the supervision of the missing individual to file the missing person's report. Other states identified medical personnel, long-term care ombudsman, a long-term care facility, cohabitants, and neighbors or close friends among those eligible to file a missing persons report in order to active an alert. Four states (Colorado, Florida, Kentucky, and Ohio) indicated that any individual can file a missing persons report in order to activate an alert.

Criteria for Activating an Alert

Once the appropriate individual has filed a missing persons report with the local law enforcement agency, the agency must review the report to determine if the state's criteria for activating an alert have been met. In addition to determining whether or not the missing person meets any age or disability criteria for activating an alert system (see section on Target Population above), all states reported additional criteria.

Table 4. Selected Criteria for Activating an Alert

State	Status is Unknown[a]	Threat to Health or Safety[b]	Sufficient Information[c]	Domiciled in or Resident of State[d]
Colorado	Yes	Yes	—	Yes
Delaware	Yes	Yes	—	Yes
Florida	Yes	Yes	Yes	—
Georgia	Yes	Yes	Yes	—
Kentucky	—	Yes	—	—
North Carolina	Yes	—	—	—
Ohio	Yes	Yes	Yes	—
Oklahoma	—	Yes	Yes	—
Rhode Island	—	Yes	Yes	—
Texas	Yes	Yes	Yes	Yes
Virginia	Yes	Yes	—	—

Source: Congressional Research Service based on correspondence with state officials between September 2008 and March 2009.

Notes: Categories based on responses to the question "What are the criteria for issuing an alert?"

a. States reported the following: the person's whereabouts are unknown; the person is believed to be missing; investigation by local law enforcement has verified or confirmed the person is missing. In Florida, the local law enforcement agency must have activated a local or regional alert and verified vehicle tag information.

b. States reported either that the person's disappearance poses a credible threat to their safety and health or that the person is in imminent danger of serious bodily injury or death.

c. States reported the following: there is sufficient information about the person's disappearance to disseminate to the public; there is enough descriptive information regarding the missing person or his/her vehicle; there is sufficient information to disseminate to the public that could assist in the investigation; or disseminating information to the public or media would assist in locating the person. In Florida, there must be a description of the vehicle and a tag number to display on the electronic highway sign.

d. States did not furnish a detailed definition of the terms domiciled in or resident of the state.

Four criteria for activating an alert that are common across the 11 states include (1) the person's status is unknown; (2) the person's disappearance poses a credible threat to his or her health or safety; (3) there is sufficient information to provide information to law enforcement agencies and/or the public about the missing individual; and (4) the person is domiciled in or a resident of the state in which they went missing. **Table 4** summarizes the presence of these four criteria by state.

States with alert systems for missing vulnerable adults have certain criteria for activating an alert that are somewhat similar across the states. Most states reported that a person's whereabouts must be unknown in order for an alert to be activated. In some states, local law enforcement have conducted a missing person's investigation and verified that the person is missing. Almost all states, the exception being North Carolina, indicated that the person's disappearance must either pose a credible threat to his or her health and safety or that the missing person is in immediate danger of serious bodily injury or death. Six of the 11 states reported that the alert may only be activated if there is sufficient information about the person's disappearance. For example, in Texas and Georgia there must be sufficient information to disseminate to the public and in Oklahoma submitting information to the public or media would assist in locating the person. Only a few states require that alerts be activated on behalf of persons who are domiciled or a resident of the state. In Colorado and Texas, the missing person must have been domiciled in the state. To activate an alert in Delaware, the missing person must be a Delaware resident.

In addition to these four criteria, states may have other criteria that must be met before an alert is activated. For example, Florida only activates statewide alerts on electronic highway signs for those individuals who are missing and believed to be driving a vehicle, thus the state first requires activation of a local or regional alert and a description of a vehicle or tag number. Florida also requires the missing person's information be entered into the Florida Crime Information Center. North Carolina requires the local law enforcement agency to report the incident to the North Carolina Center for Missing Persons. Rhode Island reported that the person must have last been seen in the state in order for an alert to be activated.

Mechanisms for Disseminating the Alert

As discussed above, one difference among states with alert systems is the designated entity responsible for activating the alert. Among the 11 states, six states (Colorado, Georgia, North Carolina, Ohio, Rhode Island, and Texas) have a lead state agency that is responsible for activating alerts at the request of a local law enforcement agency. In the remaining five states (Delaware, Florida, Kentucky, Oklahoma, and Virginia) the local law enforcement agency activates the alert locally or regionally and can seek assistance from the state law enforcement agency to disseminate the alert statewide or to another state, if necessary. For example, in Oklahoma, local law enforcement agencies activate alerts to law enforcement entities via the Oklahoma Law Enforcement Telecommunication System (OLETS), a communication system operated by the state's Department of Public Safety, which facilitates communication about missing adult alerts to law enforcement agencies throughout the state.

In general, the entity responsible for activating the alert will disseminate descriptive information about the missing person to other law enforcement entities and the public through agreements with designated media and other information outlets. States identified television, radio, newsprint, lottery terminals, electronic highway signs, and trucker alert systems among those entities involved in further disseminating information about the missing person. States reported that this descriptive information may be disseminated electronically by e-mail or by facsimile. Some states will use the National Law Enforcement Telecommunications System (NLETS) or a similar state-named system (e.g., OLETS) to disseminate information about the missing person, this may be through a "be on the lookout" message to law enforcement agencies.[16] Multiple states automatically authorize the use of electronic highway signs for dissemination of the alert, while other states use electronic highway signs on a case-by-case basis. Two states, Florida and North Carolina, reported the ability to use a reverse 911 system that leaves a recorded telephone message with information about the missing person and whom to contact with information.

Target Audiences

Once an alert has been activated and information has been disseminated to local law enforcement and the media, local law enforcement agencies in all states are asked to "be on the lookout" for the missing person and media outlets are encouraged, but not required, to provide the public with information on the missing person and their disappearance. States that post information in lottery terminals and on electronic highway signs provide information about the missing person to the public through these forms of communication. When information is disseminated to the public, information on how to contact law enforcement with tips or information is also included. States may include one or more contact numbers for the public to utilize such as the telephone number for the local law enforcement agency directing the search or the state alert system's coordinating office, emergency telephone systems such as 911 or 511, or the telephone number for state highway patrol.

Duration of the Alert

Some states impose certain conditions related to the timing and duration of an alert that has been activated, while others do not. In general, states do not have a waiting period prior to the activation of an alert. One state, Texas, requires that the activation of an alert be implemented within 72 hours of the person's disappearance. Five states (Florida, Ohio, Oklahoma, Texas, and Virginia) reported certain time constraints regarding the duration of active alerts. Oklahoma and Texas activate alerts for up to 24 hours; however, the requesting agency in Texas has the option to ask for an extension. In addition, time durations could also differ if a law enforcement agency decided to issue an alert locally or through an existing regional program. In Virginia, alerts can be activated for up to 12 hours, while Ohio evaluates the need for the alert after 48 hours and each 24 hours thereafter. The electronic highway signs in Florida are activated for six hours; however, information on the Florida Department of Law Enforcement's (FDLE) web-site can be posted as long as the person is missing. The remaining six states (Colorado, Delaware, Georgia, Kentucky, North Carolina, and Rhode Island) do not impose a time limit for the activation of alerts, but may give various stakeholders discretion regarding the duration of the alert. In Rhode Island and Delaware, the media outlets can determine how long they will broadcast the alert. Georgia will discontinue the alert at the family's discretion. North Carolina does not impose a time period for activation of the alert, but reported that alert information on electronic highway signs is activated for up to 12 hours.

Interstate Coordination

The 11 states were asked about whether they coordinated with other states to recover individuals who are believed to have crossed state lines during their disappearance. Most of the states have some mechanisms in place for coordinating with other states. Notably, most also share a border with at least one other state with an alert system.

If needed, officials said they would send information about a missing adult from their state through national or interstate law enforcement communication systems. Colorado, Florida, Georgia, Texas, and Virginia reported that they would use NLETS. Delaware would disseminate information about a missing resident to fusion centers in nearby states, which are comprised of relevant law enforcement agencies in a particular jurisdiction that share information.[17] Ohio officials said that information would be conveyed to other states through "law enforcement computer systems," but did not specify which systems. Florida, Georgia, and North Carolina indicated that their missing persons clearing houses could coordinate with clearinghouses in other states. Rhode Island reported that it would coordinate with the other state's state law enforcement agency. Officials in a few of the states noted possible constraints in reporting residents missing, since most other states do not appear to have alert systems. Some officials suggested that states without the systems could ask law enforcement officials to "be on the lookout" for a missing individual.

At least four states have requested other states (all of which are featured in the report) to activate alerts on behalf of residents (though this information was provided only by the states that were asked to activate the alert). Nearly all states, with the exception of Texas, reported that an alert could be activated on behalf of a missing individual from another state. Texas officials said that a missing senior who came from another state would not meet one of the alert criteria – that the individual is domiciled in Texas, meaning that he or she is a full-time resident of the state. However, a local law enforcement agency could coordinate a public notification response within the affected areas for an individual not domiciled in the state, if permitted by the local authorities, without requesting assistance from the state alert network. For instance, a local law enforcement agency could enlist the assistance of media, public agencies, and other local entities. Further, officials in at least four regions could seek assistance from regional alert networks which have been established to recover missing adults. As discussed above, Colorado and Delaware include residency as part of their alert criteria; nonetheless, these states indicated that an alert could be issued on behalf of an individual who is not a resident.

Finally, nearly all states require that reports of missing persons be entered into the National Crime Information Center (NCIC) Missing Person File.[18] The NCIC is used by law enforcement agencies in all states to inquire about criminal and missing person cases. For instance, if a law enforcement officer comes across a missing individual, the officer can search the NCIC database for any information about the individual that may have been entered by a law enforcement agency in that state or another state.

System Costs

All states provided data about costs related to state-level agencies that carry out (or assist in carrying out) alerts for missing adults. For states that provided detailed information, cost estimates ranged from about $40,000 to

$182,000 to operate the alert systems annually. No states provided information about any costs to local law enforcement agencies or other stakeholders that may be involved in helping to administer the alert system.

Colorado and Florida specified that the costs for implementing and administering the missing adult alert systems have been absorbed, in part, by the budget for the AMBER Alert system. Colorado additionally reported that there are ongoing costs for personnel and maintenance of both systems, but these costs were not specified. Florida reported that the administrative costs for both the AMBER and missing adult alerts include the salaries of on-call missing adult clearinghouse staff. The approximate cost is $40,000 per fiscal year.

Georgia, North Carolina, and Ohio explained that funds are not set aside specifically for their adult alert systems, but that the cost of administration is absorbed by the budgets of the agencies that administer the alerts. North Carolina estimated that the cost to the missing person's clearinghouse, the agency that administers the alert, is $125,000 annually. Officials in Ohio reported that an upgrade to their AMBER Alert and missing person alert technology will cost approximately $100,000 at some future point.

Virginia and Texas provided more detailed cost information. Texas reported costs associated with the Governor's Division of Emergency Management (GDEM) and the Texas Missing Persons Clearinghouse, which jointly administer the alert system (and does not include costs to other agencies). The approximate cost to the GDEM for coordinating the program with its existing AMBER Alert and Blue Alert[19] programs and providing training on these programs was approximately $92,000, which excludes initial operating costs. The GDEM has a coordinator to administer the alert system, along with the state's other alert systems. This position, along with ongoing costs for training and coordination activities are funded in state FY2009 through a grant ($47,280) and internal operating expenses for the GDEM ($45,000). The Missing Persons Clearinghouse, which provides investigative support to the GDEM, has two analysts dedicated to the alert system. Actual expenses, including salaries, operations, and travel for state FY2008, were approximately $90,000. In total, the approximate cost annually to Texas for the alert system is about $182,000.

Virginia officials provided cost data for the state police to activate regional or statewide alerts (local alerts are activated by local law enforcement agencies). In state FY2007, the cost was $30,000 for implementing the program, and an additional $30,000 for staff time and technology. The estimated ongoing costs are $25,000 annually. The ongoing costs are for staff time to administer the system, including handling and processing requests for the alert, activating the alert, assessing the alert after it has been activated, posting and removing information to the Virginia State Police Department missing persons website, and creating posters. According to state officials, the state will need about $50,000 to implement technology for the alert system and $45,000 annually for training, outreach, and staff support.

Delaware, Rhode Island, and Oklahoma reported that no costs for the states are associated with the alert system. This appears to be, in part, because the alerts in Delaware and Oklahoma are administered and activated primarily by local law enforcement agencies, with some assistance from the state police or department of public safety. Kentucky did not provide any funding information, which also may be due to the fact that alerts are locally managed.

Use of the System

Nearly all states, with the exception of Delaware, reported that alerts have been activated. Kentucky and Oklahoma do not keep records of alerts activated by local law enforcement agencies, but estimated that no more than 10 alerts have been activated in each state. The other eight reporting states provided the number of alerts activated, even if only at the state level, and most provided information about the outcomes of missing individuals. States reported activating between one (Rhode Island) and 82 alerts (North Carolina) as of the time they were surveyed. As previously mentioned, the number of alerts is likely affected by when the systems were implemented, the size of the state's population, and criteria for activating the alerts.

Outcomes

Most states provided some information about the circumstances around a missing person's disappearance and their recovery. All states reported that the majority of the individuals were found alive, though at least one individual was found deceased in nearly every state, except Rhode Island. Five states (Florida, North Carolina, Ohio, Texas,[20] and Virginia) indicated how the missing individuals were traveling. Florida's missing adult alert is activated only for individuals who are driving; therefore, all 32 (100%) missing individuals for whom alerts were activated were driving. In North Carolina, of the 82 alerts activated, 43 (52.4%) were on behalf of individuals who were driving and 39 (47.6%) had wandered away. Of those 39 individuals, three took a plane to another state, two were last seen on bikes, one took a bus to another state, and one took a taxi. Of the 14 individuals for whom alerts were activated in Ohio, nine (64.3%) of the individuals were driving. In Texas, of 71 alerts activated, 58 (81.7%) of the individuals were driving and 13 (18.3%) individuals wandered from their home or another location. Of the seven individuals for whom alerts were activated in Virginia, one (14.3%) was believed to have been driving. Two states (Florida and Georgia) provided information about where the missing individuals were found. Of the seven individuals in Florida who were recovered as a result of the alert system, six were located a few counties away from their home county. In Georgia, of the 78 alerts for individuals who were found, one was located in another state with family and the other 77 were located within their home city or county.

Six states (Florida, Georgia, North Carolina, Rhode Island, Texas, and Virginia) were able to report whether the alerts aided in the recovery of missing individuals.[21] Half of those states reported that the alert systems have been instrumental in recovering missing adults while the other states reported that the alerts did not help in recovery efforts. Florida officials stated that seven of 32 individuals (21.9%) were recovered based on tips provided by drivers who had seen electronic messages on the highway about the missing adults. According to officials in Georgia, the alert aided in the recovery of all individuals who were recovered alive (which was all but one individual). In Texas, of the 77 alerts activated, they contributed to the recovery of 21 senior citizens (27.3%). Rhode Island has activated one alert, and according to state officials, the alert did not assist in the individual's recovery. Officials in North Carolina reported that the alerts did not directly assist in the recovery of the missing individuals; however, family members of the missing individuals and the law enforcement agencies that recommended the alert be activated are pleased with the design of the program. Finally, Virginia officials reported that the alert did not assist in the recovery of the seven individuals who went missing and for whom alerts were activated.

DISCUSSION

This report describes the detailed findings of 11 states with active alert systems for missing adults. Findings from this study suggest that there is an existing patchwork of state alert systems with wide variation in target populations and administrative procedures for activating alerts. These systems are similar to alert systems for abducted children (AMBER Alerts), but target adults who are vulnerable to going missing due to cognitive or mental impairment, developmental or physical disabilities, and certain mental health conditions. Although the systems in each state vary, in all states either local or state law enforcement agencies are responsible for activating the alerts. Often these law enforcement agencies involve multiple stakeholders in the process of recovering those who go missing, including other local law enforcement agencies, the state highway patrol, the public through various media outlets, and the state's missing persons clearinghouse.

As the nation prepares for an aging population and likely increase in the number of individuals living in the community with cognitive impairment or other forms of disability, Congress may want to consider whether there is a role for the federal government in further developing state alert systems. For example, the federal government could provide funding to facilitate the expansion of alert systems to additional states. Similar to the federal role for state AMBER Alert programs, the federal government could assist in developing minimum guidelines for a missing adult alert system as well as provide states with technical support and training. Establishing a uniform network of state alert systems in every state could assist states and localities, in the event that a person is believed to be missing, with any necessary coordination across state lines. Further, the federal government could also play a role in assisting states with developing their systems so that data are more uniformly collected about the use and efficacy of state alert systems. Finally, the federal government could disseminate information about best practices for states looking to implement alert systems.

The following sections discuss various issues for Congress in considering the role of the federal government, if any, in state alert systems for vulnerable missing adults. These issues are: autonomy and individual rights; creating a uniform identity; training; coordination across states; efficacy of alerts; use of alerts; and support to family caregivers.

Autonomy and Individual Rights

The use of any alert system for missing adults may challenge the legal rights of an individual, in this case an adult, who may choose to go missing. Unlike the AMBER Alert program which was established to alert law enforcement and the public when a child is missing and criminal activity may be involved, it is not a crime for an adult to wander from home or purposely go missing. To attempt to balance the rights of an individual with the concerns of family members or caregivers, states with alert systems have established specific criteria that must be met in order to activate a missing adult alert. In general, states have targeted missing individuals who are particularly vulnerable due to a credible threat to the individual's health and safety. Also, as previously mentioned, timing can be a critical factor in locating individuals with cognitive or mental impairment who wander either on foot or in a vehicle and may be without basic provisions or medicine, or exposed to the elements for extended periods. Concerns about violating an individual's privacy with respect to filing a missing person's report appear to outweigh the perceived benefits among various stakeholders including family members, law enforcement officials, and policymakers. While states were not explicitly asked for information about whether reports of missing persons were credible, state officials in one state, Texas, indicated that all alerts activated by the state were based on legitimate reports of missing vulnerable seniors. In general, states felt the criteria they had established contained appropriate safeguards to ensure that missing persons were in fact missing due to a cognitive impairment or some other disabling condition.

Creating a Uniform Identity

The popularity of state AMBER Alert systems appears to provide a platform for states to develop their missing adult alerts. Naming the missing adult alert system as a Senior, Silver, or Gold Alert may be an attempt by states to create a "brand" identity for the system similar to that of state AMBER Alerts. For example, three states use the word "Senior" in the title of their system: Colorado's Missing Senior Citizen Alert Program; Rhode Island's Missing Senior Citizen Alert Program; and Virginia's Senior Alert System. Another four states refer to their alert systems as a "Silver Alert," which is likely a reference to an older person (i.e., someone with grey or silver hair). However, the senior or silver reference may also be misleading in that it may not accurately describe the target population for these alert systems. In some states with a "Silver Alert" or "Senior Alert" system, alerts can also be activated on behalf of missing persons aged 18 to 59. Other states refer to their alert systems as Gold or Golden Alert or Missing Adult Alert. These named programs tend not to specify age criteria for activating an alert. The use of a name to create a specific brand identity for the alert system could also serve to distinguish the alert system from AMBER Alerts or other types of alerts.

Further, creating a brand identity could be done to prompt law enforcement entities and the public to respond to the alert in a specific way that may be different from the response for other types of alerts. Similar to AMBER Alert, the federal government may want to consider a uniform name or identity for state alert systems for missing vulnerable adults to assist states in implementing alert systems, coordinating alerts across states, and educating various stakeholders about the system.

Training

Most states with alert systems reported that law enforcement agencies have been trained on the procedures for activating missing adult alerts in their respective states. However, in some states where a local law enforcement agency activates the alert, it was not known whether there was uniform training at the local level. In addition, states were not asked the extent to which these alert systems train law enforcement and other public safety officials in techniques to assist in recovering persons with cognitive or mental impairments. Some advocates argue that specific training on Alzheimer's disease and related dementia can be effective in both identifying and recovering these individuals in the event they go missing.[22] Moreover, persons who wander away from home may easily attract the attention of law enforcement through auto accidents or erratic driving, indecent exposure, shoplifting, and other deviant behavior. Often these individuals can not think, act, or communicate in a way that can assist them. However, proper training in identifying and communicating with an individual who has a mental or cognitive impairment can help to ensure that these individuals are returned safely to their home. Pending legislation (H.R. 632 and S. 557) to assist states develop and coordinate missing adult alert systems would include a training component where a federal coordinator, working in collaboration with the Administration on Aging and the Missing Alzheimer's Disease Patient Alert program, would provide training opportunities and educational resources to law enforcement and other entities.

Coordination Across States

Some states with alert systems reported that they might have difficulty coordinating with another state that lacks a similar system. States may also have challenges coordinating with states that have alert systems with different criteria for activating an alert. Although state and local governments have taken the lead in implementing alert systems, the federal government could play a role in coordinating efforts when a missing individual is believed to have crossed state lines as well as assist in the development of formal agreements or protocols for the use of interstate alerts.

The federal government could model any policies to coordinate across state lines on the AMBER Alert program, which provides training and technical assistance to states on a number of issues related to abducted children. This training addresses how jurisdictions, including those in different states, can work together to recover children who are abducted, among other topics. Through conference and training exercises, state AMBER Alert coordinators, state and local law enforcement agencies, and other stakeholders have opportunities to meet and exchange ideas, which may further facilitate coordination. In addition, the DOJ has issued recommended guidelines for activating AMBER Alerts to encourage states and localities to adopt similar alert criteria. Existing legislation (H.R. 632 and S. 557) that would create a similar network of state missing adult alert systems seeks to provide greater coordination between states for missing adult cases by establishing a Silver Alert Coordinator position at the DOJ. The purpose of the position is to help establish voluntary guidelines for states in developing Silver Alert plans that will promote compatible and integrated Silver Alert systems throughout the United States.

Effectiveness of Alerts

It is not clear how effective state alert systems are in recovering missing vulnerable adults. At least a few of the states with alert systems did not maintain detailed outcomes data on the alerts that had been activated to date, and many could not report whether the alert was useful. In states where alerts are activated at the local level, aggregating data on the outcomes of these alerts may be more complicated than in states that have a designated agency at the state level that activates alerts. Furthermore, tracking outcomes from alerts is an administrative task that may require additional technology and resources, which states may not have the funding to support. Further, only three (Florida, Georgia, and Texas) of six states that reported whether the alerts were effective could say for certain that the reports aided in the recovery in the missing individual. For Georgia, the alert aided in all cases, while in Florida and Texas the alerts aided in fewer than 30% of all cases. The federal government could play a role in developing guidelines for data collection and outcomes measures as well as assisting states with developing technology and infrastructure necessary for reporting on the use and effectiveness of their alert systems.

USE OF ALERTS

Some states expressed that overuse of alerts for vulnerable adults could desensitize the public to alerts in general, including AMBER Alerts.[23] State officials in Oklahoma and Virginia, both of which administer missing adult alert systems locally with some state-level involvement, commented that the Emergency Alert System, which may be used for AMBER Alerts, should not be used for missing adult alerts so that the public does not become desensitized to AMBER Alerts (note that the FCC does not allow the system to be used for purposes related to missing persons except for abducted children). Officials in Virginia further stated that the EAS is best for missing children because they are more likely to have been removed from their communities, whereas missing vulnerable adults tend to wander on foot in close proximity to the place they were last seen. This is consistent with the Alzheimer's Association's statement that most wandering adults with the disease are found within one mile of their home.[24] State officials concerned about using scarce law enforcement resources to recover missing vulnerable adults raised the issue of whether activating the alert system was the best use of these resources. Some states have expressed concern as to whether the alert systems should be used only in select circumstances and/or for select populations. In response to these concerns, states may choose to activate alerts regionally or statewide only in the case where an individual is believed to be driving, given that they can readily travel outside of their community.

SUPPORT TO FAMILY CAREGIVERS

Alert systems for vulnerable adults can assist local and state law enforcement agencies in the recovery of a missing adult; however, they often fail to address the circumstances that led to the person's disappearance. As previously mentioned, it is not uncommon for people with cognitive impairment resulting from Alzheimer's disease to wander away from home and become lost. According to the Alzheimer's Association, six out of ten people with Alzheimer's disease will wander during the course of the disease, sometimes frequently.[25] Some state and local law enforcement agencies have integrated the Alzheimer's Association's Safe Return program into their routines. Other law enforcement agencies are working in their communities to provide electronic monitoring services for certain individuals who are susceptible to going missing close to home and may not be visible to the public.[26] Missing alert systems for vulnerable adults could benefit from developing formal linkages with these programs, where they exist, and assist with disseminating information to the community about accessing these programs. Proposed legislation would authorize funding for grants to states and local governments to carry out programs that provide electronic monitoring services to elderly individuals that could assist in their recovery if they go missing.[27]

In the event that a state activates an alert for a missing vulnerable person and that individual is recovered alive, state alert systems may benefit from engaging community social services agencies or, in the case the individual is a senior, partnering with state units on aging and local area agencies on aging, funded under the Older Americans Act. These agencies or organizations could conduct caregiver assessments with the aim of preventing future wandering behavior. The caregiver assessment process could identify and link appropriate services and support for family caregivers such as back-up support, in cases of emergency, counseling, or respite care. Many of these services are already available to caregivers through federal funding that supports the National Family Caregiver Support Program (NFCSP).[28] Caregiver assessments would also elicit information about the caregiver's health, willingness to provide care, and training and support needs. Through the assessment process family caregivers could learn about the resources available to them in their communities including the Alzheimer's Association's Safe Return Program or Project Lifesaver International, Inc., which has developed a program to track missing vulnerable adults through electronic technology.

CONCLUSION

State alert systems for missing vulnerable adults appear to be an emerging trend, with alert systems developed in at least 11 states. As a result, Congress is considering legislation that would provide the federal government with a role in assisting states to develop these systems nationwide. Most states with existing alert systems have modeled their program after the AMBER Alert program. All state systems target persons with cognitive or mental impairments; however, there is wide variation in the specific target population and procedures for activating alerts. While states will continue to be faced with the challenge of balancing individual rights with efforts that can assist the most vulnerable of residents, states may benefit from federal efforts that could facilitate interstate coordination for missing persons believed to have crossed state lines. In addition, federal efforts could model the federal role in developing state AMBER Alerts systems by providing states with minimum guidelines, technical assistance, and training. State alert systems may also benefit from coordinating with existing federal, state, and local initiatives that can assist in locating vulnerable adults that go missing. In the event that the alert system assists in recovering a missing vulnerable adult, family caregivers may benefit from referral to the Safe Return Program, funded in part by federal appropriations under the Missing Alzheimer's Disease Patient Alert grant, or Project Lifesaver International, Inc. These alert systems could also educate and assess family caregivers about the needs of vulnerable adults and provide linkages to available community resources in an effort to prevent future wandering behavior.

APPENDIX A. QUESTIONS FOR STATE OFFICIALS

Table A-1. Questions on Alert Systems for Missing Adults Submitted to State Officials

Questions by Category
A. Authorizing Legislation and Statutory Citation 1. What legislation authorized the alert system? What is the statutory citation, if any?
B. Reason for Developing Alert System 1. What was the impetus for developing an alert system for missing adults (i.e., media attention, governor's direction, legislative action, other)?
C. Administration of the Alert System 1. Name the entity or entities that have the responsibility for administering the missing adult alert system (e.g., state police, state department of safety, missing person's clearinghouse, other).
D. Target Population 1. Who is the target population for the missing adult alert system (e.g., age, disability type, other)?

Questions by Category
E. Process for Activating an Alert 1. Which entities may take a report of a missing person (e.g., law enforcement (specify whom), missing person clearinghouse, other)? Is there a standard intake form? If so, can you provide a copy of this form? 2. Which individual is authorized to make the report of the missing individual (e.g., spouses, parents, caretakers, legal guardians)? 3. What are the criteria for issuing an alert? 4. Which entity issues the alert? 5. If the alert criteria are met, is the entity required to issue the alert (mandatory) or is issuing the alert at the discretion of that entity (voluntary)? 6. Is there a waiting period requirement in order to issue an alert? 7. To whom is the alert issued (e.g., law enforcement, media, state government agencies, and/or the public, etc.) and how are these alerts issued? 8. Does the entity coordinate with the state department of transportation about placing information about the alert on an electronic sign on the highway? 9. What are law enforcement, media, and/or the public expected to do when they receive the alert? For example, are law enforcement agencies in a particular area asked to search for the missing individual and/or lookout for a car that the individual is believed to be driving? 10. If the alert is issued to the public, how can they inform appropriate officials that the missing individual has been located? 11. For how long may an alert be issued?
F. Association with AMBER Alert The U.S. Congress is interested in understanding the relationship between the missing adult alert system and the state's AMBER Alert system for missing children. Please describe the relationship, if any, between these two alert systems, including: 1. Are both alert systems administered by the same agency? 2. Do both types of alerts use the same process described above, including the same technology? If not, how is the alert system for missing adults different than the AMBER Alert system?
G. Interstate Coordination The U.S. Congress is interested in learning about how your state's missing adult alert system coordinates alerts with other states when a person is believed to have crossed state lines. Please describe the procedures, if any, for coordinating alerts across state lines: 1. Does your state have a process for informing other states that a missing adult for whom an alert has been issued in your state may be located in another state ? If so, please describe this process (include information such as the number of times the state has requested an alert to be issued, states coordinated with, circumstances for issuing the alert, outcomes of these missing persons cases)? 2. Can your state issue an alert on behalf of a missing adult who is a resident of

Table A-1. (Continued)

Questions by Category
another state, but believed to be in your state? If so, please describe this process (include information such as the number of times an alert has been issued in your state on behalf of another state, states coordinated with, circumstances for issuing the alert, outcomes of these missing persons cases)?
H. Program Costs 1. What were the costs, if any, associated with implementing the alert system? Please provide a dollar value for the most recent fiscal year available. Specify whether the fiscal year is federal (i.e., October 1 through September 30) or state (indicate the start and end dates for the state fiscal year). 2. What are the costs associated with ongoing administration of the alert system? Please provide a dollar value for the most recent fiscal year available. 3. If possible, please specify what the ongoing administrative costs are associated with (e.g., technology, labor, other)? Please provide a dollar value for each.
I. Use of Alert System The U.S. Congress is also interested in the extent to which the missing adult alert systems have been utilized and the extent to which data is available on outcomes from use of the system. 1. In which month and year was the alert system implemented? 2. How many alerts have been issued since the system was started and through the most recent date available? 3. How many were recovered alive? Deceased? 4. In how many cases did an alert aid in the recovery of an individual, regardless of whether the person was recovered alive or deceased? 5. In cases where the individual was recovered due to the alert, which entity located that individual? How far was the individual from his/her residence or last known location? 6. In how many cases was the missing individual believed to have: Alzheimer's disease or other forms of dementia? Other mental impairments? If the missing individuals did not have Alzheimer's disease/dementia or mental impairments, what was the reason they were believed to be vulnerable? 7. In how many cases was the missing individual believed to be driving?
J. Other 1. Does the state require law enforcement agencies to add information about missing adults (for whom an alert has been issued) to the FBI National Crime Information System's Missing Person File or to any state missing persons database? 2. Does the state provide education and training to law enforcement or other stakeholders (e.g., radio and TV broadcasters, department of transportation officials, etc.) about the alert system? If so, which entity provides this training, and for whom is the training provided? What type of training is provided?

Source: Prepared by the Congressional Research Service.

Appendix B. Detailed Tables of State Programs

Table B-1. Colorado: Alert System for Missing Adults State refers to system as "Colorado Missing Senior Citizen Alert Program"

Topics Inquired About	Response by State
Authorizing Legislation and Purpose for Developing Alert System	In 2006, Governor Bill Owens signed S.B. 06-057 establishing a missing alert program for missing senior citizens and missing persons with developmental disabilities system, and requiring the Colorado Bureau of Investigation (CBI) to implement the program (see Section 24-33.5-415.8 of the Colorado Revised Statutes). The CBI subsequently implemented a program for missing senior citizens, known as the "Missing Senior Citizen Alert Program."a The impetus for developing the program, as specified in S.B. 06-507, is that recovering missing seniors within the first few hours of their disappearance is vital, and the program can aid in recovering these individuals. The program was implemented in April 2006.
Administration	The Missing Senior Citizen Alert Program is administered by the CBI, in coordination with local law enforcement agencies. The alert is issued by the CBI at the request of a local law enforcement agency.
Training on and/or Education About the Alert System	The CBI offers training and disseminates information about the system through brochures and the CBI website. Entities that receive the training include public, media, law enforcement, and the Alzheimer's Association, among other entities.
Association with AMBER Alert	Both the AMBER Alert system and Silver Alert system are administered by the same agency, the CBI. The same process is used to issue alerts on behalf of abducted children and missing adults, except that an AMBER Alert is distributed more widely and it is broadcast through the Emergency Alert System (EAS).
Target Population	The target population is missing senior citizens with a verified impaired mental condition.
Reporting the Missing Person	Any individual may file a missing person report for the missing senior. Upon notice that a senior citizen is missing, local law enforcement agencies are required to verify that the senior citizen is missing and that he or she has an impaired mental condition. To verify an impaired mental

Table B-1. (Continued)

Topics Inquired About	Response by State
	condition, a family member (or close friend, caregiver, doctor, or medical facility) must sign a statement stating that the missing person is mentally impaired. Upon receiving a request made by a local law enforcement agency, the CBI first must verify information about the identity of the law enforcement agency, confirm that the law enforcement agency has received the signed statement that the missing senior has an impaired mental condition, and verify that the information meets the definition of "missing senior citizen" (see below). The alert may then be issued. CBI corresponds with the requesting law enforcement agency to determine what steps the agency has taken to further their investigation. The local law enforcement agency has discretion in determining whether to request the CBI to issue the alert.
Information About Missing Persons Submitted to Databases	The CBI requests that law enforcement agencies enter information into the federal National Crime Information Center (NCIC) Missing Person File if the information has not already been entered.
Criteria for Issuing Alert	The following definition of a missing senior citizen must be met to activate an alert. A missing senior citizen is a person: • whose whereabouts are unknown; • whose domicile is in Colorado; • who is 60 years of age or older; • who has a verified impaired mental condition; and • whose disappearance poses a credible threat to the safety and health of the person, as determined by local law enforcement.
Disseminating Alert	The alert is issued to law enforcement agencies and the public through the media, including radio stations, television stations, and other media outlets. CBI advises that the media may include information about the missing senior's name, last known location, mode of transportation, events leading to the senior's disappearance, and his or her health and safety. Highway signs are used to display information only if the missing person is believed to be driving a vehicle. Law enforcement agencies are notified via National Law Enforcement Telecommunications

Table B-1. (Continued)

Topics Inquired About	Response by State
	System (NLETS) and a "be on the lookout" alert.
Timing of Alert	There is no waiting period for issuing an alert. An alert remains active until the individual is located. The CBI is responsible for cancelling the alert, and will notify media outlets if the missing senior has been found or at the end of the broadcasted notification period.
Expected Respo-nse by Law Enforcement and/or Public	The public is asked to call 911 or local law enforcement with information. Law enforcement agencies contact the CBI with information.
Interstate Coordination	The CBI notifies law enforcement in surrounding states through NLETS. If the CBI had reason to believe the missing individual traveled to another state, the agency would contact the other state's law enforcement agency. If a missing individual from another state went missing in Colorado and the circumstances of their disappearance meet the alert criteria, the CBI would issue the alert.
System Costs	The implementation costs were absorbed by resources for the AMBER Alert system. There are ongoing costs associated with personnel and maintenance of the notification systems.
Use of Alert System	From approximately April 2006 through January 2009, the CBI issued eight alerts.
Outcomes	Of the eight individuals for whom alerts were issued, all were recovered alive. In all cases, the individual had an impaired mental condition based on the state's criteria for issuing an alert.

Source: Congressional Research Service based on correspondence with state officials in January 2009 and review of Section 24-33.5-415.8 of the Colorado Revised Statutes and accompanying rules and regulations.

a. The state did not provide information about any alert program for persons with developmental disabilities.

Table B-2. Delaware: Alert System for Missing Adults State refers to system as "Gold Alert Program"

Topics Inquired about	Response by State
Authorizing Legislation and Purpose for Developing Alert System	In 2008, Governor Ruth Ann Minner signed S.B.l 227 establishing the Delaware Gold Alert Program (see Sections 8580-8583 of the Delaware Code). The impetus for developing the program was based on interest by members of the legislature. The program was implemented in July 2008.
Administration	The Gold Alert program is administered by local law enforcement agencies, in coordination with the Delaware State Police's Information and Analysis Center (DIAC) and the media. The investigative law enforcement agency issues the alert in cooperation with the DIAC.
Training on and/or Education About the Alert System	Delaware State Police troopers have been informed of the Gold Alert procedures and protocols through a monthly roll call training session. State officials are unsure what type of training local law enforcement officers receive about the alert.
Association with AMBER Alert	The Delaware State Police is the only law enforcement entity authorized to disseminate an AMBER Alert. If another agency is investigating an abducted child case, it must contact the Delaware State Police to request an alert. The Gold Alert does not have the same criteria as the AMBER Alert. The investigating law enforcement agency determines if the Gold Alert is warranted, and is responsible for activating it. Law enforcement agencies follow the same protocols for disseminating press releases about the missing individual as they would for an abducted child. However, unlike the Gold Alert, the AMBER Alert is broadcast on billboards, roadway signs, and through the media. Based on an agreement with the Broadcasters Association, media outlets must broadcast an AMBER Alert.
Target Population	The target population is missing persons with a disability, missing senior citizens who are persons age 60 or older, and missing suicidal persons who are persons whose statements, actions, or conduct indicate that the person may voluntarily cause or inflict self-harm.
Reporting the Missing Person	Persons that are related to or live with the missing person may report missing person cases. If medical personnel

Table B-2. (Continued)

Topics Inquired about	Response by State
	have sufficient information about the missing person, they may file a report. If all criteria are met, the investigating law enforcement agency is to issue the alert.
Information About Missing Persons Submitted to Databases	Information about the missing person must be entered into the National Crime Information Center (NCIC) and the Delaware Justice Information System (DELJIS).
Criteria for Issuing Alert	The following criteria must be met for issuing an alert: • the person's whereabouts are unknown; • the person is a resident of Delaware; and • the disappearance poses a credible threat to the health or safety of the person, as determined by the investigating law enforcement agency. In all cases, the investigating officer will verify the disability or impairment. If the officer determines that the person is in fact disabled or impaired, the alert will be issued. Proof from a medical authority that the person is disabled or impaired is not required.
Disseminating the Alert	The law enforcement agency that is investigating the missing person sends an alert to all enforcement agencies and designated media outlets in Delaware. Alerts are issued through a standard electronic press release from the investigating law enforcement agency via email and/ or fax. The DIAS can disseminate the information to all area law enforcement agencies and surrounding states' fusion centers (which are comprised of relevant law enforcement agencies in a particular jurisdiction that share information). Local media entities have discretion in broadcasting the alerts to the public. According to state officials, law enforcement agencies and local media have a strong working relationship, and officials would expect the media to broadcast the alert. The alert includes information that may assist in the safe return of the missing person. Electronic highway signs are not utilized in the program.
Timing of Alert	There is no waiting period for issuing an alert and there is no time limit on how long the Gold Alert remains active. Media outlets determine how long they will broadcast the alert to the public.

Table B-2. (Continued)

Topics Inquired about	Response by State
Expected Response by Law Enforcement and/or Public	The public is asked to call 911 or their local law enforcement agency with information about the individual.
Interstate Coordination	If the CBI had reason to believe the missing individual traveled to another state, the DIAC would disseminate information about the missing person to surrounding states' fusion centers. Also, as part of standard investigative procedure, if the missing person is believed to be in another law enforcement agency's jurisdiction, that agency would be contacted by the investigating law enforcement agency, and information would be shared. If Delaware had credible and reliable information that a missing person from another state may be within the state, an alert would be issued on that person's behalf.
System Costs	There are no costs associated with the program.
Use of Alert System	From approximately July 2008 through January 2009, local law enforcement agencies did not issue any alerts.
Outcomes	The state did not report on outcomes. As stated above, no alerts had been issued as of the time we inquired about the alert system.

Source: Congressional Research Service based on correspondence with state officials in January 2009 and review of Sections 8580-8583 of the Delaware Code.

a. It is unclear whether accompanying rules and regulations have been promulgated.

Table B-3. Florida: Alert System for Missing Adults State refers to system as "Florida Silver Alert Plan"

Topics Inquired About	Response by State
Authorizing Legislation and Purpose for Developing Alert System	In 2008, Governor Charlie Crist signed Executive Order 08-211 establishing the Florida Silver Alert Plan. The impetus for creating the alert was the passage of Chapter 2008- 162 (signed by the governor on June 17, 2008), which amended Section 937.021 of the Florida Statutes. The amended law requires local law enforcement to establish procedures for taking reports of missing adults, and to allow reports of missing adults to be made to the

Table B-3. (Continued)

Topics Inquired About	Response by State
	Florida Department of Law Enforcement's (FDLE) Missing Endangered Persons Information Clearinghouse (MEPIC). As specified in Executive Order 08-211, Florida's senior population is growing and the state needed to implement a standardized system to aid in the search of senior citizens who go missing. The alert system was implemented in October 2008.
Administration	The Silver Alert Plan is administered by the FDLE/ MEPIC, in coordination with local law enforcement agencies, the Florida Department of Elder Affairs, the Florida Department of Transportation, and the Florida Department of Highway Safety (which includes the Florida Highway Patrol). The FDLE/MEPIC activates the alert on highway road signs if specified criteria are met (see below). In addition, local law enforcement agencies may issue a Silver Alert locally, in coordination with the media.
Association with AMBER Alert	AMBER Alerts are carried out by the FDLE/M EPIC. The Silver Alerts are initiated by local law enforcement, and may involve the FDLE/M EPIC. The process for the Silver Alerts is not exactly the same as the process for AMBER Alert. The Silver Alerts require that local law enforcement agencies issue media statements and notify other law enforcement. The FDLE/M EPIC is responsible for activating only the road signs, and placing information on their home webpage. AMBER Alerts are administered by the state. FDLE/M EPIC carries out every step of the alert, such as the media notifications via radio and television, law enforcement, road signs, lottery machines, websites, the National Center for Missing and Exploited Children (NCMEC), and other notification systems.
Training on and/or Education About the Alert System	When funding is available, training to law enforcement and transportation officials will be conducted by the FDLE/M EPIC. Executive Order 08-211 specifies that the Florida Department of Elder Affairs is to actively share information about the existence of the plan with key advocacy groups, services providers, and other organizations or agencies serving the state's senior citizen population.

Table B-3. (Continued)

Topics Inquired About	Response by State
Target Population	The target population is a missing person age 60 or older who has an "irreversible deterioration of intellectual facilities (i.e., dementia)," as verified by law enforcement officials, and under extraordinary circumstances for a missing person age 18 to 59 who has an "irreversible deterioration of intellectual faculties."
Reporting the Missing Person	Any individual is permitted to make a report of a missing person, as long as the report is credible. The local law enforcement agency may issue an alert locally, or request that an alert be issued on highway signs through the FDLE/ MEPIC, which will issue the alert if the criteria are met.
Information About Missing Person Submitted to Databases	If a credible missing person report is made to a law enforc-ement agency, the agency is required under Florida Statute 937.02 1 to enter information into the federal National Crime Information Center (NCIC) Missing Person File and the Florida Crime Information Center (FCIC).
Criteria for Issuing Alert	The following criteria must be met to activate an alert statewide on highway signs, at the request of a local law enforcement agency: • The missing person must be 60 years or older and there must be a clear indication that the individual has an irreversible deterioration of intellectual facilities (i.e., dementia), as verified by law enforcement, or under extraordinary circumstances when a person age 18 to 59 has an irreversible deterioration of intellectual faculties and law enforcement has determined the missing person lacks the capacity to consent; and that the use of dynamic message road signs may be the only possible way to rescue the missing person. • Local law enforcement has already activated a local or regional alert by contacting media outlet in their and/or surrounding jurisdiction(s). • The law enforcement agency's investigation must conclude that the disappearance poses a credible threat to the person's welfare and safety. • If a vehicle is involved and the statewide messaging system is requested, there must be a description of the vehicle and a tag number to display on Florida Department of Transportation dynamic message signs.

Table B-3. (Continued)

Topics Inquired About	Response by State
	• The local law enforcement agency must verify vehicle tag information and have entered the missing person into the FCIC and issued a statewide "be on the lookout" to other law enforcement/911 centers.
Disseminating the Alert	The FDLE/MEPIC notifies the general public through road signs and the FDLE website. The investigating agency may contact the FDLE/M EPIC to activate the road signs if the alert criteria are met. Road signs are used only if a vehicle is involved (and the individual meets other criteria). The FDLE/M EPIC provides the Silver Alert vehicle information to the Florida Department of Transportation. Separately, local law enforcement agencies have different strategies for notifying the public, which may include contacting the media and using a type of reverse 911 calling system (through the organization, A Child is Missing, Inc.) with a recorded message telling local residents about the alert. Local law enforcement agencies issue a "be on the lookout" alert through a system for law enforcement agencies, and notify their local media however they deem appropriate.
Timing of Alert	A waiting period is not required before issuing an alert on the road signs. The road signs are activated for six hours. The information on the FDLE website is posted as long as the person is missing.
Expected Response by Law Enforcement and/or Public	Law enforcement are asked to be on the lookout for the individual and their vehicle. The media is requested to publicize the information on the missing individual and the public is asked to notify law enforcement if the missing person or vehicle is seen. Any information is to be reported to the investigating law enforcement agency, a local law enforcement agency via 911, or the Florida Highway Patrol (*347).
Interstate Coordination	Because Silver Alerts have not been instituted in every state, the state has not yet addressed how requests will be handled when it is suspected that the missing person crossed state lines. However, Florida law enforcement agencies can inform agencies in another state through the use of the federal National Law Enforcement Telecommunications System (NLETS). The FDLE/MEPIC

Table B-3. (Continued)

Topics Inquired About	Response by State
	may also contact AMBER Alert coordinators in states with Silver Alert systems to request activation for a missing adult. The FDLE/MEPIC will activate road signs for an out-of-state resident if the Silver Alert criteria are met. Florida has had one Silver Alert request from Georgia, involving a missing senior who was known (through use of credit cards) to be in Florida. The missing incident met the activation criteria. Road signs were in the process of being activated when the missing person was located.
System Costs	Funds used to maintain the AMBER Alert system are used for the Silver Alert plan. The administrative costs provide for analysts of both the Silver Alert and AMBER Alert systems to be on call year around. The approximate cost to FDLE is $40,000 per fiscal year (July 1, 2008 through June 30, 2008).
Use of Alert System	From approximately October 2008 through December 2008, the FDLE issued 32 Silver Alerts on highway signs.
Outcomes	In order to issue the statewide alert on the road signs, an individual must be believed to be driving (and meet other criteria). Of the 32 alerts issued, 31 individuals were recovered alive and one was found deceased. All were driving, and in at least 30 of the 32 cases, it was believed that the missing individual suffered from a form of dementia or Alzheimer's disease. Road sign activation aided in the recovery of seven individuals. The local law enforcement agency recovered these individuals based on tips from persons who read the highway signs. One individual was located within the same county. The other six individuals were located a couple of counties away from where they went missing. According to the state, the alerts on the road signs aided in the recovery of seven individuals.

Source: Congressional Research Service based on correspondence with state officials in January 2009 and review of Executive Order 08-211 and Section 937.021 of the Florida Statutes.

Table B-5. (Continued)

Topics Inquired About	Response by State
	mental or cognitive impairment and who disappearance poses a credible threat to the health or safety of the person, as determined by the local law enforcement agency.)
Timing of Alert	There is no time limit on how long the Gold Alert remains active. The search for the missing person must be undertaken for a minimum of two hours.
Dissemination Alert	The law enforcement agency that is investigating the missing person sends an alert to the local emergency management director, local search and rescue coordinator, local media outlets, and KYEM. The methods for disseminating the alerts vary, but multiple methods are encouraged. Local officials may activate the alerts through electronic message boards. Media outlets are not required to broadcast the alert, although they typically provide a description of the person and contact information. Local law enforcement officials and the media are sensitive to privacy issues.
Expected Response by Law Enforcement and/or Public	The public is asked to call a number to provide any information about the individual.
Interstate Coordination	Kentucky does not have a system for coordinating with other states if a missing person from the state crosses state lines, but would be willing to work with these other states. Further, if a missing individual was believed to have crossed into Kentucky from another state, KYEM would issue a statewide media alert about the individual.
System Costs	*State officials provided a response of "unknown."*
Use of Alert System	From approximately July 2009 through February 2009, local law enforcement agencies have issued alerts for approximately 15 individuals.
Outcomes	Of the 15 individuals for whom alerts were issued, three were found deceased. The alert assisted in the recovery of about seven to nine individuals.

Source: Congressional Research Service based on correspondence with state officials in March 2009 and review of Chapter 039F00 of the Kentucky Revised Statutes.

Table B-6. North Carolina: Alert System for Missing Adults State Refers to System as "Silver Alert Program"

Topics Inquired about	Response by State
Authorizing Legislation and Purpose for Developing Alert System	In 2007, North Carolina Governor Mike Easley signed H.B. 38 establishing a Silver Alert program (see Section 43B-499.8 of the North Carolina General Statutes). The system was developed in response to anticipated increases in the population of individuals with dementia and cognitive impairment. The system was implemented on December 19, 2007.
Administration	The Silver Alert program is administered by the North Carolina Center for Missing Persons (NCCMP), an agency within the North Carolina Department of Crime Control and Public Safety, in coordination with local law enforcement agencies and the North Carolina Department of Transportation. The NCCMP is the only agency that can activate the Silver Alert System and will do so only at the request of an investigating law enforcement agency.
Association with AMBER Alert	The North Carolina Center for Missing Persons administers both the AMBER Alert system and Silver Alert system. The Silver Alert was modeled on the AMBER Alert. However, the Emergency Alert System (EAS) is used only for AMBER Alerts.
Training on and/ or Education About the Alert System	Training is provided to law enforcement agencies and non-profit organizations by NCCMP staff when requested.
Association with AMBER Alert	The North Carolina Center for Missing Persons administers both the AMBER Alert system and Silver Alert system. The Silver Alert was modeled on the AMBER Alert. However, the Emergency Alert System (EAS) is used only for AMBER Alerts.
Target Population	The target population is individuals, of any age, who are believed to have dementia or other forms of cognitive impairment.
Reporting the Missing Person	A parent, spouse, guardian, legal custodian, or person responsible for the supervision of the missing individual may make the report. A local or state law enforcement agency takes the report of a missing person. The responding law enforcement agency must first investigate

Table B-6. (Continued)

Topics Inquired about	Response by State
	the missing person case and determine if the criteria are met for issuing a Silver Alert. If the Silver Alert criteria are met, law enforcement agencies then call the NCCMP to request a Silver Alert. The law enforcement agency also fills out a form that includes information about the reporting law enforcement agency, date of incident, and description of the individual, among other information. The reporting party must sign an Author-ization to Release Information before any information will be released to the public and media. If the criteria are met, the alert must be issued by the NCCMP.
Information About Missing Persons Submitted to Databases	The law enforcement agency immediately enters the information into the federal National Crime Information Center (NCIC) Missing Person File.
Criteria for Issuing Alert	The following criteria for a missing person must be met to activate a Silver Alert: • the person is believed to be suffering from dementia or other cognitive impairment, as determined by the person making the report; • the person is believed to be missing – regardless of circumstance; • a legal custodian of the missing person has submitted a missing person's report to the local law enforcement agency where the person went missing; and • law enforcement reports the incident to the NCCMP.
Timing of Alert	The NCCMP is to "make every effort to disseminate the [alert] as quickly as possible" (North Carolina Statutes 1 43.B-499.8). No agency may observe any waiting period. The alert may be activated as long as needed until the person is located. The electronic highway signs, discussed below, are activated for 12 hours.
Dissemination Alert	The alert is issued and relayed to all appropriate law enforcement agencies, the media, the public, North Carolina State Highway Patrol Communications Centers, and the executive management of the North Carolina Department of Crime Control and Public Safety. Law enforcement issues a statewide "be on the lookout"

Table B-6. (Continued)

Topics Inquired about	Response by State
	bulletin to all law enforcement agencies and provides a 24-hour phone number to receive lead calls during the investigation. If the individual is wandering or has walked away, law enforcement also activates phone calls in the immediate area using a type of reverse 911 calling system (through the A Child is Missing Program) with a recorded message telling local residents about the alert. The NCCMP posts and updates information about the alert on the department's website, notifies the local media about the missing person, and requests the North Carolina Depart ment of Transportation to activate highway message signs in cases where a vehicle is used. The highway signs are activated statewide if the individual is driving a motor vehicle.
Expected Response by Law Enforcement and/or Public	Law enforcement agencies in the affected area as well as statewide are sent the "be on the lookout" bulletin. Anyone is expected to call 911 or highway patrol in the event of a sighting. The public is asked to contact the NCCMP, dial 911, or call the highway patrol with any information regarding the missing individual. The requesting agency's phone number is also provided. When highway signs are activated, motorists are notified about the missing individual and directed to call 511 for further information. The recorded message on 511 is available for 48 hours.
Interstate Coordination	The state informs contiguous states through the use of a "be on the lookout" bulletin through the NCIC. If necessary, the NCCMP contacts other missing person clearinghouse managers in other states. Alerts may be issued on behalf of a resident of another state. The missing person report is taken by the law enforcement agency that has jurisdiction over where the person was last known to be. The agency calls the NCCMP and requests a Silver Alert. For example, the NCCMP activated an alert on behalf of an individual who was following his wife in a separate vehicle as they were traveling home to Florida. The man was thought to be missing in the Sanford, North Carolina area. The wife reported him missing and the Sanford Police Department took the report and requested the Silver Alert. The man later turned up safe at his home in Florida.

Table B-6. (Continued)

Topics Inquired About	Response by State
System Costs	The General Assembly did not appropriate funding to implement and operate the Silver Alert system. The program costs are absorbed by the NCCMP budget. The NCCMP estimates that the cost to operate the program annually is approximately $125,000.
Use of Alert System	From December 19, 2007 through October 15, 2008, the NCCMP issued 82 alerts.
Outcomes	Of the 82 individuals for whom alerts were issued, 73 were found safe, seven were found deceased, and two were still missing. Further, 52 individuals were reported to have Alzheimer's disease or dementia and 30 individuals were reported with some other cognitive impairment. In 43 cases, the individual was driving a motor vehicle. In 39 cases, the individual wandered away on foot. Of those 39 individuals, three took a plane to another state, two were last seen on bikes, one took a bus to another state, and one took a taxi. According to state officials, the alert may not have been the single reason for finding the missing individual, but in every case, the state reported that it has brought attention to the individual who needs help. The state reported that it has not evaluated the circumstances in which the individuals went missing.

Source: Congressional Research Service based on correspondence with state officials in October 2008 and review of Section 43B-499.8 of the North Carolina General Statutes.

Table B-7. Oklahoma: Alert System for Missing Adults State refers to system as "Silver Alert System"

Topics Inquired about	Response by State
Authorizing Legislation and Purpose for Developing Alert System	In 2006, the Oklahoma House of Representatives adopted House Resolution 1055, which authorizes the creation of a Silver Alert System. Pursuant to the adoption of Resolution 1055, local law enforcement agencies, in partnership with the Department of Public Safety (DPS), implemented the system in June 2007.
Administration	The system is administered by local law enforcement agencies, in coordination with DPS and the media. The

Table B-7. (Continued)

Topics Inquired About	Response by State
	local law enforcement agency issues the alert, and can seek assistance from DPS, which houses the Oklahoma Enforcement Telecommunications System (OLETS), a communication system that can be used to inform other law enforcement agencies about missing adult alerts and other matters.
Association with AMBER Alert	The AMBER Alert system is administered by the Department of Public Safety, and the Silver Alert system is administered by local law enforcement agencies in cooperation with DPS. The two systems use similar technology. For AMBER Alerts, the local law enforcement agency completes a form on an OLETS terminal and it is sent to a central law enforcement communications facility, operated by the Department of Public Safety, in Oklahoma City. The AMBER Alert is then sent to television, radio, and print media. The Silver Alert uses the same system; however, when the form is completed, the reporting agency sends the alert directly to the media and appropriate law enforcement agencies. Further, AMBER Alerts can be broadcast through the Department of Transportation's electronic signs on the highway. The Emergency Alert System (EAS) may be used only for AMBER Alerts. According to state officials, the EAS may not be appropriate for Silver Alerts; too many alerts may make the public complacent, and in turn, the AMBER Alert program may not be as effective.
Training on and/or Education About the Alert System	Training is provided to law enforcement personnel that operate the Oklahoma Law OLETS terminals, by the state's Council on Law Enforcement and Education Training and select personnel from various law enforcement agencies in the state. According to state officials, information may also be provided to local law enforcement agencies through their training academies.
Target Population	The target population is individuals with a proven mental or physical disability. According to state officials, the Silver Alert system is primarily used to recover senior citizens. However, Resolution 1055 is silent on any age criteria.
Reporting the Missing Person	Spouses, parents, caretakers, legal guardians, or medical personnel, or individuals who come across the missing

Table B-7. (Continued)

Topics Inquired About	Response by State
	person may report that an individual is missing. Local and state law enforcement agencies take the report. At the request of a local law enforcement agency, the reporting party is responsible for providing the appropriate information about the condition of the individual. These agencies must first investigate the missing person case and determine if the criteria are met for issuing a Silver Alert. If the criteria are met, law enforcement agencies complete a form in the state's law enforcement database to initiate the alert. The form includes information about the reporting law enforcement agency, date of incident, and description of the individual, among other information. Issuing the alert is at the discretion of the agency.
Information About Missing Persons Submitted to Missing Person Database	Local law enforcement agencies are not required to enter information into the federal National Crime Information Center (NCIC) Missing Person File or other law enforcement databases for missing persons.
Criteria for Issuing Alert	The following criteria must be met to activate a Silver Alert: • the person must have a proven mental or physical disability, as determined by a caretaker or medical personnel; • there is reason to believe that the person is in imminent danger of serious bodily injury or death; and • disseminating information to the general public or media would assist in locating the person. At the request of a local law enforcement agency, the caregiver, medical personnel or family member would be responsible for providing the appropriate information about the condition of the individual. The law enforcement agency would determine if this information is adequate. Oklahoma using OLETS. The information is sent electronically via OLETS to the media. The public is made aware of the alert by television, radio, and print media. Electronic signs, including those operated by the Department of Transportation, are not activated when a Silver Alert is issued.

Table B-7. (Continued)

Topics Inquired About	Response by State
Dissemination Alert	Silver alerts may be issued to law enforcement agencies locally, regionally, or statewide, and to the media. These alerts are issued to all law enforcement agencies in
Timing of Alert	There is no waiting period to issue the alert. The alert may be activated for up to 24 hours.
Expected Response by Law Enforcement and/or Public	The agencies are requested to broadcast the information to their officers, and the media may alert the public. Any tips and information are to be reported to the local law enforcement agency that issued the alert or to 911.
Interstate Coordination	Law enforcement officials may announce the alert to officials in other states through the National Law Enforcement Telecommunication System (NLETS), using OLETS. If the missing individual from Oklahoma is (or believed to be) in another state or en route to another state, information in the Silver Alert will be sent to that state via OLETS. If Oklahoma receives information that an individual from another state who is the subject of a Silver Alert, is believed to be in Oklahoma, that information would be sent via OLETS to the law enforcement agencies and the media in Oklahoma.
System Costs	According to state officials, there were little, if any, costs to DPS associated with developing the Silver Alert system.
Use of Alert System	Local law enforcement agencies issue the alerts and maintain records about the alerts issued and whether individuals were recovered. This information is not submitted to the Department of Public Safety or any other state entity. State officials estimated, based on anecdotal information, that six alerts were issued from approximately June 2007 through September 2008.
Outcomes	The state did not report on outcomes. As discussed above, information about the individuals for whom alerts are issued is not systematically collected.

Source: Congressional Research Service based on correspondence with state officials in September and October 2008 and review of Oklahoma House Resolution 1055.

Table B-8. Ohio: Alert System for Missing Adults
State refers to system as "Missing Adult Alert System"

Topics Inquired About	Response by State
Authorizing Legislation and Purpose for Developing Alert System	In 2008, Governor Ted Strickland signed Senate Bill 87 establishing the Ohio Missing Adult Alert system (see Section 5502.522 of the Ohio Revised Code). The alert was developed in response to several incidents of missing adults throughout the country and Ohio that involved older individuals or individuals with mental impairments. The system was implemented in June 2008.
Administration	The alert system is administered by the Bureau of Criminal Identification and Investigation, within the Ohio Attorney General's office, in coordination with local law enforcement agencies, Ohio State Highway Patrol, other state agencies, and the media. Together, these agencies make up the Ohio AMBER Alert Steering Committee, which developed the AMBER Alert and Missing Adult Alert systems. The Ohio Attorney General's Office or the Ohio State Highway Patrol are the only agencies that can activate an alert, and will do so at the request of an investigating law enforcement agency.
Association with AMBER Alert	The Ohio AMBER Alert Steering Committee has oversight over the AMBER Alert and Ohio Missing Adult Alert systems. The processes and tools are similar for both programs. The same technology is used for both programs; however, the Emergency Alert System (EAS) is used only for AMBER alerts.
Training on and/ or Education About the Alert System	Law enforcement agencies are trained by members of the AMBER Alert Steering Committee. Training covers the program criterion and activation process.
Target Population	The target population is individuals ages 65 or older, or adults ages 18 or older with a mental impairment. "Mental impairment" means a "substantial disorder of thought, mood, perception, orientation, or memory that grossly impairs judgment, behavior, or ability to live independently, or provide self-care as certified by a licensed physician, psychiatrist, or psychologist" (Section 5502.522(G)(3) of the Ohio Revised Code).

Table B-8. (Continued)

Topics Inquired About	Response by State
Reporting the Missing Person	Local and state law enforcement agencies take reports of a missing person. These agencies must first investigate the missing person case and determine if the criteria are met for issuing an alert. Requesting an alert is at the discretion of the law enforcement agency. A report can be made to local law enforcem-ent by any individual. Issuing the alert is at the recommendation of the local law enforcement agency and at the discretion of that agency, the Ohio Attorney General's office, or Ohio State Highway Patrol.
Information About Missing Persons Submitted to Database	Information must be entered into the federal National Crime Information Center (NCIC) Missing Person File as part of the local law enforcement agency's request to issue the alert.
Criteria for Issuing Alert	The following criteria must be met to activate an alert: • the local investigative law enforcement agency confirms the individual is missing; • the individual is 65 years of age or older, or has a mental impairment; • the disappearance of the individual poses a credible threat of immediate danger of serious bodily harm or death to the individual; and • there is sufficient descriptive information about the circumstances surrounding the individual's disappearance to indicate that activation of the alert will help locate the individual. Individuals who identify the person as missing are not required to attest that the person is missing due to their condition; however, they may provide prescriptions or other medical paperwork to verify that the individual is under the care of a licensed medical professional.
Dissemination Alert	The alert is issued to all appropriate law enforcement agencies, the media, truckers, the Ohio Lottery Commission, Ohio Outdoor Advertising Association, and the public. Email and fax messages are sent throughout the state to media outlets. The information is posted on electronic billboards and Ohio Department of Transport-ation signboards in the local area of interest, and a Truckers Alert system is activated for truckers in the state.

Table B-8. (Continued)

Topics Inquired About	Response by State
	The Ohio Lottery posts the information on lottery terminals. Alerts are also issued on electronic signs managed by the Ohio Department of Transportation and the Ohio Outdoor Advertising Association.
Expected Response by Law Enforcement and/or Public	The Ohio Attorney General's Office coordinates special response teams and programs to assist in the search for the missing person. Law enforcement may also form their own search teams. Teams may help in direct search, media relations, victim services and case investigation. Law enforcement and the public are asked to be observant in finding the individual. The media's role is to disseminate information to the public. Any tips and information are to be reported to a toll-free telephone number, local law enforcement, or 911.
Timing of Alert	There is no waiting period to issue the alert and no set time limit for an alert to be issued. The Ohio Attorney General's Office, in consultation with the local law enforcement agency, evaluates the need for the alert after 48 hours and each 24 hours thereafter.
Interstate Coordination	Alert information is shared with adjacent states through law enforcement computer systems. Ohio has not requested an alert on behalf of an adult who is believed to be in another state. Ohio can issue alerts on behalf of adults who reside in other states but are believed to be in the state. Ohio's criteria for issuing an alert must be met before an alert may be issued. To date, no states have requested Ohio to issue an alert.
System Costs	A budget was not developed to implement the alert system, and costs have been absorbed by the state agencies on the AMBER Alert Steering Committee. Those agencies have not developed any estimates on the cost to implement the system. The precise ongoing costs are unknown. Labor and other costs vary based on the number of alerts issued, duration of the alerts, and state employees involved in issuing the alert. In the future, the agencies expect to pay for improved notification software, estimated at \$100,000 for both AMBER and Missing Adult Alerts.
Use of Alert System	From approximately June 2008 through September 2008, the Ohio Attorney General's Office and the Ohio State

Table B-8. (Continued)

Topics Inquired About	Response by State
	Highway Patrol issued 14 alerts.
Outcomes	Of the 14 individuals for whom alerts were issued, 13 were found alive and one was found deceased. Seven of the missing individuals had Alzheimer's disease and/or dementia; four had mental health issues; and two had medical issues and were ages 65 or older. Nine of the individuals were driving. According to state officials, the alerts did not directly assist in the recovery of the missing individuals; however, family members of the missing individuals and the law enforcement agencies that recommended the alert be activated are pleased with the design of the program.

Source: Congressional Research Service based on correspondence with state officials in September 2008 and review of Section 5502.522 of the Ohio Revised Code.

Table B-9. Rhode Island: Alert System for Missing Adults State refers to system as "Missing Senior Citizen Alert Program"

Topics Inquired About	Response by State
Authorizing Legislation and Purpose for Developing Alert System	In 2008, the Rhode Island General Assembly passed S7048 and H7048 creating the Rhode Island Missing Senior Citizen Alert program (See Sections 42-28-3.3 and 42-28- 3.4 of the Rhode Island Code). The bills were effective without the governor's signature in July 2008. Private agencies that care for the senior population with mental health concerns sought and received support from members of the state legislature who introduced the bill that was eventually passed into law after several years trying. The program was implemented in September2008.
Administration	The alert program is administered by Rhode Island State Police, in coordination with local law enforcement agencies, the Rhode Island Broadcasters Association (RIBA), and other agencies such as the Rhode Island Department of Transportation. The Rhode Island State Police issues the alert to media outlets and the local law enforcement agency conducts the investigation.

Table B-9. (Continued)

Topics Inquired About	Response by State
Training on and/ or Education About the Alert System	The Rhode Island State Police provided training to all local law enforcement agencies about the program.
Association with AMBER Alert	The Rhode Island State Police administers both AMBER Alerts and the Missing Senior Citizen Alert program. The agency issues the AMBER Alert, while RIBA issues the Missing Senior Citizen Alert. Further, the agency is more directly involved with the investigation of AMBER Alerts and handles inquiries from the media and the public about these alerts. The local law enforcement agency is responsible for handling these types of inquiries for Missing Senior Citizen Alerts.
Target Population	The target population is for a missing person whose whereabouts are unknown, who is a resident of Rhode Island, who is age 60 or older, who has an impaired mental condition.
Reporting the Missing Person	The missing senior citizen's family, legal guardian, long-term care ombudsman, or long- term care facility where such person resides, may report the person missing. The reporting party must provide the appropriate document-ation showing that the individual has an impaired mental condition. If all criteria are met, the investigating law enforcement agency requests the Rhode Island State Police to issue the alert through RIBA.
Information About Missing Persons Submitted to Databases	Local law enforcement agencies are not required to enter information into the federal National Crime Information Center (NCIC) Missing Person File or other law enforcement databases for missing persons.
Criteria for Issuing Alert	The following criteria must be met for issuing an alert: • the person is age 60 or older; • the person has an impaired mental condition supported by documentation; • the circumstances surrounding the person's disappearance poses a credible threat to their safety and health; • the person must have last been seen in Rhode Island; and • enough descriptive information is available for the

Table B-9. (Continued)

Topics Inquired About	Response by State
	• missing person and/or his or her vehicle. In all cases, the investigating law enforcement agency will verify the mental condition.
Disseminating the Alert	Upon request by the Rhode Island State Police, RIBA disseminates the alert to media outlets, that are members of the organization. These media outlets have discretion in broadcasting the alerts to the public. Electronic highway signs maintained by the Department of Transportation may be activated on a case-by-case basis. The alert includes information that may assist in the safe return of the missing person.
Timing of Alert	There is no waiting period for issuing an alert and there is no time limit on how long the alert remains active. Media outlets determine how long they will broadcast the alert to the public.
Expected Response by Law Enforcement and/or Public	The public is asked to call 911 or their local law enforcement agency with information about the individual.
Interstate Coordination	If the Rhode Island State Police had reason to believe the missing individual traveled to a bordering state, the agency would disseminate information about the missing person to the state police agency. If a missing person from another state was last seen in Rhode Island, the investigation would be handled as if the individual was from Rhode Island. The state has not had to request alerts for residents nor has it issued alerts for residents of other states.
System Costs	There are no costs associated with the program.
Use of Alert System	From approximately September 2008 through February 2009, the Rhode Island State Police issued an alert on behalf of one individual with a mental condition who was recovered alive.
Outcomes	The individual for whom an alert was issued was not driving. The alert did not assist in the recovery of the individual.

Source: Congressional Research Service based on correspondence with state officials in March 2009 and review of Sections 42-28-3.3 and 42-28-3.4 of the Rhode Island Code.

Table B-10. Texas: Alert System for Missing Adults State refers to system as "Silver Alert Network"

Topics Inquired about	Response by State
Authorizing Legislation and Purpose for Developing Alert System	In May 2007, Governor Rick Perry signed S.B. 1315, creating the Texas Silver Alert Network. (see Sections 411.381-411.389 of the Texas Government Code). As specified in S.B. 1315, the impetus for the law was based on concerns that senior citizens with Alzheimer's disease or other mentally debilitating diseases wander from their residences and may die if not found. The legislation stated that "[a]n alert system similar to the AMBER Alert Program could help to locate these persons before any harm happens to them." The system was implemented in September 2007.
Administration	The Silver Alert Network is administered by the Governor's Division of Emergency Management (GDEM), with the investigative support of the Department of Public Safety's (DPS) Missing Person's Clearinghouse and in coordination with local law enforcement agencies. The GDEM issues the alert at the request of a local law enforcement agency. A Steering Committee and After-Action Review Board - comprised of law enforcement agencies, other government agencies, and other stakeholders -provide recommendations to DPS about the Silver Alert program, but have no direct authority to administer the program.
Training on and/or Education About the Alert System	The GDEM offers training to law enforcement agencies statewide about the Silver Alert Network. In addition, information about the Silver Alert is provided to public, private and local governmental entities through briefings, conferences, and workshops. An existing Online AMBER Alert Course, currently available to law enforcement and the public, may be used in the future to provide information about the Silver Alert.
Target Population	The target population is senior citizens, age 65 or older, who are domiciled in Texas, and have a diagnosed impaired mental condition.
Reporting the Missing Person	An immediate family member, caretaker, or legal guardian may report that an individual is missing. In some cases, the report may be filed by a neighbor or close friend who

Table B-10. (Continued)

Topics Inquired About	Response by State
	notices the person is missing. Local and state law enforcement agencies take reports of a missing person. These agencies must first investigate the missing person case and determine if the criteria are met for issuing a Silver Alert (see below). If the criteria are met, law enforcement agencies then fax a Silver Alert Request Form to the GDEM and follow up with a phone call. The form includes information about the reporting law enforcement agency, date of incident, and description of the individual, among other information. The alert is issued at the request of an investigating law enforcement agency and after DPS has confirmed that a request for activation meets the criteria. If the alert criteria are met, the alert must be issued.
Information About Missing Persons Submitted to Databases	Information about the missing person must be entered into the federal National Crime Information Center (NCIC) Missing Person File before an alert is activated.
Criteria for Issuing Alert	The following criteria must be met to activate the Texas Silver Alert Network: • the missing person is 65 years of age or older; • the senior citizen is domiciled in Texas; • the senior citizen has a diagnosed impaired mental condition, and their disappearance poses a credible threat to the senior citizen's health and safety (law enforcement requires the family or legal guardian of the missing senior citizen to provide documentation from a medical or mental health professional of the senior citizen's condition); • an investigation has confirmed that the senior citizen's disappearance is due to his/her impaired mental condition, and alternative reasons for his/her disappearance have been ruled out; • the Silver Alert request is within 72 hours of the senior citizen's disappearance; and • there is sufficient information available to disseminate to the public that could assist in locating the senior citizen.

Table B-10. (Continued)

Topics Inquired About	Response by State
Dissemination Alert	The GDEM issues alerts to the public through primary and participating media outlets; the Texas Department of Transportation; the Texas Lottery Commission; and the Independent Bankers Association of Texas. Local primary media stations are provided with a fax notification. Media participation is voluntary. The Texas Lottery Commission places Silver Alert information on their electronic scrolling signs, billboards, and tickets (as applicable). The Independent Bankers Association of Texas, depending on the technology available at each institution, can place Silver Alert information within their lobbies and drive-through locations, along with electronic scrolling signs and billboards. Local, state and federal law enforcement agencies are also provided alert advisories through the Texas/National Law Enforcement Telecom-munications System (TLETS/NLETS). (As part of training to law enforcement entities, they are encouraged to coordinate with local media when Silver Alerts are activated.) In addition, the GDEM maintains an email notification database for those entities (such as a government entity, including the military, or business) that wish to provide notification to the public. Highway signs are activated by the Texas Department of Transportation only if accurate vehicle information is available *and* it is confirmed that the senior citizen was driving the vehicle at the time of the disappearance.
Timing of Alert	There is not a waiting period to issue the alert. An alert may be issued for up to 24 hours. The requesting agency has the option to request extensions, granted upon review by the GD EM.
Expected Response by Law Enforcement and/or Public	Law enforcement and the public are encouraged to look for the missing senior citizen. Media outlets (which may voluntarily participate) are encouraged to provide Silver Alert information to the public. The GDEM provides state network partners with information about the missing senior citizen, along with vehicle information if it is available. The public is encouraged to contact the appropriate law enforcement agency. The number of the agency is provided.

Table B-10. (Continued)

Topics Inquired About	Response by State
Association with AMBER Alert	The GDEM administers both AMBER and Silver Alerts. The systems operate independently, although training on the Silver Alert system has been incorporated into the existing AMBER Alert coordination and training program. (Coordination refers to those activities used to facilitate review of alerts, planning, peer-training, and strengthening communication between network partners and other participating entities.) Texas' 17 regional AMBER Alert programs are managed and operated independently of the Texas Silver Alert Network. These programs employ a multitude of local and regional resources to recover abducted children. The GDEM supports communication, peer-training, and networking with all Texas regional AMBER Alert programs through meetings and workshops. Four of the regional AMBER Alert programs have incorporated missing senior advisories within their operations, and some regional AMBER Alert programs coordinate AMBER Alerts with local counties in nearby states. The GDEM process for receiving Silver Alert requests and informing the public about the alert is similar to the process for AMBER Alerts, except that the Emergency Alert System (EAS) is used only for AMBER Alerts. In addition, AMBER Alerts are distributed through the National Center for Missing and Exploited Children (NCMEC)'s Secondary Distribution Notification System, which notifies participating law enforcement agencies, public service entities, internet and wireless providers, trucking companies, restaurant chains, and electronic billboard companies, among other entities; and to Beyond Missing.com, a program that distributes information about the alert through fax and email.
Interstate Coordination	When an individual is believed to be in another state, the GDEM routes a message about the Silver Alert through the National Law Enforcement Telecommunications System (N LETS) to the other state's law enforcement point of contact. The GDEM collects statistics on the operational aspects of an alert, such as the number of requests and activations. It does not collect investigative case data, which could include information about whether the missing individual is believed to be in another state. The legislation

Table B-10. (Continued)

Topics Inquired About	Response by State
	authorizing the Silver Alert Network indicates the missing senior citizen must be domiciled within Texas; however, local law enforcement and media could still coordinate a public notification response within the affected areas about an individual who is not domiciled in the state, without activating the Silver Alert Network.
System Costs	The following costs are associated with the GDEM and the state's missing person clearinghouse (and does not include costs to other agencies). The approximate cost to the GDEM for coordinating the program with its existing AMBER Alert and Blue Alert programs and providing training on these programs was at least $92,000 (this does not include initial operating costs). The GDEM has a coordinator to administer the alert system, along with the state's other alert systems. This position, along with ongoing costs for training and coordination activities are funded in state FY2009 through a grant ($47,280) and internal operating expenses for the GDEM ($45,000). The Missing Persons Clearinghouse, which provides investigative support to the GDEM, has two analysts dedicated to the alert system. Actual expenses, including salaries, operations, and travel for state FY2008, were approximately $90,000.
Use of Alert System	From September 1, 2007, through January 11, 2009, the GDEM issued 77 alerts for missing senior citizens.
Outcomes	Of the 77 individuals for whom alerts were issued, 71 were found alive and four were found deceased; 58 individuals were driving. According to state officials, the alert contributed to the recovery of 21 senior citizens (27.3%). As required by the alert activation criteria, the missing senior citizen must have a diagnosed impaired mental condition. No alerts were found to have been falsely reported. The GDEM collects statistics on the operational aspects of an alert, such as the number of requests and activations. It does not collect investigative case data, which would include detailed information about the circumstances around an individual's disappearance.

Source: Congressional Research Service based on correspondence with state officials in January 2009 and review of Sections 411.381-411.389 of the Texas Government Code.

Table B-11. Virginia: Alert System for Missing Adults State Refers to System as the "Virginia Senior Alert System"

Topics Inquired About	Response by State
Authorizing Legislation and Purpose for Developing Alert System	In 2007, Governor Tim Kaine signed H.B. 2372 creating the Virginia Senior Alert system (see Sections 15.2-1718.1 and 52-34.4 - 52-34.6 of the Code of Virginia). The system was created with the purpose of modeling similar efforts underway in other states. The system was implemented in July 2007.
Administration	The Senior Alert system is administered by local law enforcement agencies, in coordination with the Virginia Missing Person Information Clearinghouse, within the Virginia State Police Department; Attorney General's office; and the media. The alerts are issued locally by local law enforcement agencies, and regionally and statewide by the Virginia State Police.
Association with AMBER Alerts	The Virginia State Police Department issues all AMBER Alerts and issues regional and statewide Senior Alerts. The media is informed in the same way about the alerts, through email and facsimile. The state has a website for law enforcement agencies to request AMBER alerts. According to the state, funding is not available to build a similar website for Senior alerts. Further, the Emergency Alert System (EAS) is used only for AMBER Alerts. According to the state, the EAS may not be appropriate for Senior Alerts. Most, if not all, seniors who have been reported missing in Virginia travel on foot in close proximity to the place they were last seen. The state has explained that using EAS is more effective for AMBER Alerts because a child abduction usually happens quickly, and there is the high risk of death or serious physical injury to the child. In cases of missing seniors, the state would rather the media to report frequently about the individuals, and for search teams to begin their rescue efforts as soon as possible.
Training on and/or Education About the Alert System	The Virginia State Police train local law enforcement agencies about the system and activation process. This training covers the criteria for activation and the activation process. The Attorney General's Office has provided similar information to the public in formal presentations.

Table B-11. (Continued)

Topics Inquired About	Response by State
Target Population	The target population is individuals ages 60 years or older who suffer a cognitive impairment to the extent that he or she is unable to provide care to himself or herself without assistance from a caregiver. A cognitive impairment refers to Alzheimer's Disease or other forms of dementia.
Reporting the Missing Person	A report can be made to a law enforcement agency by any caretaker. A caretaker can attest that the individual is missing and meets the qualifying medical criteria; however, the law enforcement agency that takes the report of the missing individual determines if this information is accurate and the person's condition is suitable for the alert. Local and state law enforcement agencies take reports of a missing person. These agencies must first investigate the missing person case and determine if the criteria are met for issuing a Senior Alert, make the request (to the Virginia State Police, if needed), and complete accompanying request forms. The law enforcement agency (local or the Virginia State Police) has the discretion to issue the alert.
Entity that Issues Alert	Information about the missing person must be entered into the federal National Crime Information Center (NCIC) Missing Person File before an alert is activated.
Criteria for Issuing Alert	The following criteria must be met to activate a Senior Alert: • the person is 60 years old or older; • the person has a cognitive impairment that renders him or her unable to provide care to himself or herself without assistance (including a diagnosis of Alzheimer's disease or dementia); • the person's whereabouts are unknown; and • the person's disappearance poses a credible threat (as determined by a law enforcement agency) to his or her health or safety.
Dissemination of Alert	The alert is issued by local law enforcement agencies (for local alerts) or the Virginia State Police (for regional or statewide alerts) to other appropriate law enforcement agencies, the media, and the public. The Virginia State Police notifies radio and television media about the alert through email and facsimile. In turn, the media may inform the public. The Virginia Missing Persons Clearinghouse

Table B-11. (Continued)

Topics Inquired About	Response by State
	posts and updates information about the alert on the Virginia State Police Department's Senior Alert website and where appropriate, creates posters for the missing individuals. The state does not typically issue alerts through electronic signs on the highway or other locations, and would only use the signs if the missing person is believed to be in a car. If alerts were issued on electronic signs, these signs would be those managed by the Virginia Department of Transportation, and where available, the Lamar Advertising Company, which owns signs in the state.
Expected Response by Law Enforcement and/or Public	Law enforcement agencies and the public are asked to be observant in finding the individual. The media are not required to issue an alert about the missing individual. The law enforcement agency that initiated the alert is required to provide phone number for tips and leads, and this number must be staffed at all times.
Timing of Alert	There is no waiting period to issue the alert; however, the law enforcement agency must first determine that the individual is, in fact, missing and not accounted for at all possible locations. An alert may be issued for up to 12 hours.
Interstate Coordination	The state has not requested another state to issue an alert, but would use the National Law Enforcement Telecom System (NLETS) to transmit information about an alert. Virginia can issue alerts on behalf of adults who reside in other states but are believed to be in Virginia. However, Virginia's criteria for issuing an alert must be met before an alert may be issued, and the alert would be issued from the Virginia State Police. North Carolina requested the state to issue an alert for a missing North Carolina resident, which was activated. The individual was found deceased in North Carolina.
System Costs	The approximate costs to implement the program were \$30,000, for staff time (\$15,000) and technology (\$15,000) in state FY2007 (July 1-June 30). The estimated ongoing costs are \$25,000 annually. The ongoing costs are for staff time to administer the system, including handling and processing requests for the alert, activating the alert, assessing the alert after it has been issued, posting and

Topics Inquired About	Response by State
	removing information to the Virginia State Police Department missing website, and creating posters. The state will need about $50,000 to build technology for the alert system and $45,000 annually for training, outreach, and staff support.
Use of Alert System	From approximately July 2007 through September 2008, the Virginia State Police issued seven alerts.
Outcomes	Of the seven individuals for whom alerts were issued, five were found alive and two were found deceased. All had Alzheimer's disease or another form of dementia, and one was believed to have been driving. Most, if not all, traveled on foot in close proximity to the place they were last seen. According to the state, the alerts did not directly assist in the recovery of the missing individuals.

Source: Congressional Research Service based on correspondence with state officials in September 2008 and review of Sections 15.2-1718.1 and 52-34.4 - 52-34.6 of the Code of Virginia.

End Notes

[1] A similar version of the bill (H.R. 6064) in the 110th Congress was passed by the House on September 17, 2008.

[2] Alzheimer's disease is the most common form of dementia and it is estimated that as many as five million Americans have the disease. While memory loss is one symptom of Alzheimer's disease, other symptoms may include being disoriented to time and place. For instance, a person with Alzheimer's disease may become lost in an otherwise familiar place, such as their neighborhood or community, they may forget where they are or how they got there. For further discussion of Alzheimer's disease, see CRS Report RL32970, *Biomedical Advances in Alzheimer's Disease*, by Michele M. Schoonmaker and Laura B. Shrestha.

[3] Ashlen Anderson, "Public Policy Responses to Wandering Behavior," *Issue Kit*, Alzheimer's Association, September 2006, p. 2.

[4] For further discussion of the federal role, see CRS Report RL34616, *Missing Adults: Background, Federal Programs, and Issues for Congress*, by Adrienne L. Fernandes.

[5] Among the nearly 4,000 adults reported missing to NCMA over about an approximately three-year period, about 45% had a diagnosed medical condition that required care or medication; and 35% had a mental illness or diminished mental capacity, which includes general depression, Post Traumatic Stress Disorder (PTSD), bipolar disorder, schizophrenia, attention deficit (hyperactivity) disorder, autism, and other genetic conditions. The balance had Alzheimer's disease or related dementia (about 8%), alcohol or chemical dependency (about 7%), or another unspecified disability (about 5%). Detailed data are not available for characteristics other than disabilities.

[6] These states were mentioned as having missing adult alert programs in news articles and policy publications, including Ben Schmitt, "Silver Alerts Could Help Pinpoint Missing Seniors' Location," *USA Today*, July 8, 2008; Kelly Wilkicki, "Silver Alerts Sound the Alarm when

Certain Seniors Go Missing," *National Conference of State Legislatures*, vol. 29, no. 516 (May 27, 2008); Kathy G. Miller, "Long-Term Care: Facility Quality and Safety," Health Policy Tracking Service, Sept. 2008; National Center for Assisted Living, "NCAL Focus," American Health Care Association, Washington, DC, Aug. 2006.

[7] For the purposes of this analysis, CRS selected those states with active alert programs. Therefore, Louisiana was the only state not selected because, according to state officials, the alert system had been authorized but not yet implemented. Thus, sufficient information to describe how Louisiana's alert system operated was not available at the time of this report. CRS also identified four states—California, New York, Pennsylvania, and West Virginia—that have introduced legislation to implement similar alert programs in the last three years.

[8] The U.S. Census Bureau defines four different regions: Northeast, Midwest, South, and West. States in the Northeast region include Maine, New Hampshire, Vermont, Massachusetts, Rhode Island, Connecticut, New York, New Jersey, and Pennsylvania; states in the Midwest region include Ohio, Indiana, Illinois, Michigan, Wisconsin, Minnesota, Iowa, Missouri, North Dakota, South Dakota, Nebraska, and Kansas; states in the South region include Delaware, Maryland, the District of Columbia, Virginia, West Virginia, North Carolina, South Carolina, Georgia, Florida, Kentucky, Tennessee, Alabama, Mississippi, Arkansas, Louisiana, Texas, and Oklahoma; states in the West region include Montana, Idaho, Wyoming, Colorado, New Mexico, Arizona, Utah, Nevada, Washington, Oregon, California, Alaska, and Hawaii.

[9] Most, if not all, states have clearinghouses that serve as a repository for information about missing persons. These clearinghouses are often operated by the state's law enforcement agency.

[10] Texas also has 17 regional AMBER Alert programs, four of which have incorporated missing senior advisories as part of their operations.

[11] For further information, see CRS Report RL34050, *Missing and Exploited Children: Background, Policies, and Issues*, by Adrienne L. Fernandes.

[12] U.S. Department of Justice, Office of Justice Programs, *Report to the Congress on AMBER Alert*, July 2005, http://www.amberalert.gov/newsroom/pdfs/05_amber_report.pdf.

[13] For further information, see U.S. Department of Justice, *Secondary Distribution of AMBER Alerts*, http://www.amberalert.gov/secondary_distribution.htm.

[14] For further discussion, see CRS Report RS21453, *Amber Alert Program Technology*, by Linda K. Moore.

[15] Congressional Research Service correspondence with the FCC in February 2009.

[16] NLETS is an international computer-based message switching system that links together state, local, and federal law enforcement and justice agencies for the purpose of exchanging information. For further information, see International Justice and Public Safety Information Sharing Network, *NLETS: The International Justice & Public Safety Network*, http://www.nlets.org/WhoWeAre.aspx.

[17] For further information, see CRS Report RL34070, *Fusion Centers: Issues and Options for Congress*, by John Rollins.

[18] The NCIC is a federal computerized index with data on crimes and locator files for missing and unidentified persons, operated by the Federal Bureau of Investigation (FBI). Colorado was the only state that suggested that reporting missing adults to the NCIC is not mandatory. The state reported that the Colorado Bureau of Investigation requests, and does not appear to require, that law enforcement agencies enter information about a missing individual.

[19] Blue Alerts provide notification about offenders who have harmed law enforcement officials.

[20] Although not requested, Texas also reported that no alerts were found to have been falsely reported.

[21] Officials in North Carolina did not say whether the alerts aided in the recovery of the missing person, but said that at minimum, the alerts brought attention to the individual.

[22] Ashlen Anderson, "Public Policy Responses to Wandering Behavior," *Issue Kit*, Alzheimer's Association, September 2006, p. 2.

[23] As noted by the Alzheimer's Association, repeated alerts for those that are prone to going missing could have the effect of desensitizing the public to any alerts—for abducted children and/or vulnerable adults. Ashlen Anderson, "Public Policy Responses to Wandering Behavior," *Issue Kit*, Alzheimer's Association, September 2006, p. 3.

[24] Ibid, p. 1.

[25] Ibid, p. 1.

[26] This technology was developed by Project Lifesaver International, a nonprofit organization that administers the Project Lifesaver program. Project Lifesaver uses a personalized wristband that emits a signal to track individuals prone to going missing, such as those with Alzheimer's disease and children with cognitive disabilities. The wristband is worn by the client continuously. When family members or caregivers report to the designated Project Lifesaver agency—typically a local law enforcement or first responder agency—that the client is missing, a local search and rescue team responds to the wanderer's area to search using a mobile locator tracking system.

[27] S. 557 also authorizes the DOJ, after consulting with the Department of Health and Human Services (HHS), to create the Sammy Kirk Voluntary Electronic Monitoring Program. The program would award grants to state and local governments to carry out programs that provide electronic monitoring services to elderly individuals that would assist in their recovery if they go missing. The legislation proposes to fund the program $2 million for each of FY2010 through FY2014 for these services. Note that the companion legislation, H.R. 632, does not contain provisions related to electronic monitoring.

[28] For further information on federal programs that can assist family caregivers, see CRS Report RL34123, *Family Caregiving to the Older Population: Background, Federal Programs, and Issues for Congress*, by Kirsten J. Colello.

In: Adults Gone Missing
Editor: Thomas S. Cabrera
ISBN: 978-1-62100-085-3

Chapter 2

MISSING ADULTS: BACKGROUND, FEDERAL PROGRAMS, AND ISSUES FOR CONGRESS*

Adrienne L. Fernandes-Alcantara

SUMMARY

Adults may go missing due to choice, an abduction, foul play, a mental or physical disability, or a natural catastrophe, among other reasons. Although no accurate estimates exist of the number of missing adults, the Federal Bureau of Investigation (FBI) reported that as of January 1, 2011, nearly 50,000 missing adult cases were pending in the National Crime Information Center (NCIC) system, a federal computerized index with data on crimes and locator files for missing and unidentified persons. Certain adults are particularly vulnerable to missing episodes; for example, those with dementia are at risk for wandering. Adults who engage in high-risk behaviors, including involvement in gang activity, may also be more prone to going missing.

Unlike children, adults have the legal right to go missing under most circumstances. As a result, families of missing adults may receive limited assistance from state and local law enforcement entities in recovering their loved ones. The federal government has not been involved in assisting law enforcement entities with missing adult cases in the same way it has with

* This is an edited, reformatted and augmented version of a Congressional Research Service publication, report RL34616, dated May 27, 2011.

missing children cases. Further, cases of missing children and young adults under the age of 21 must be reported to the NCIC, while reporting missing adults to the database is voluntary. In recent years, however, the federal government has increasingly played a role in (1) preventing certain types of missing adult incidents and (2) working to recover adults who go missing, including those who are deceased and for whom only remains can be found.

Recognizing the needs of a growing aging population, Congress authorized funding for the Missing Alzheimer's Disease Patient Alert program under the Violent Crime Control and Law Enforcement Act of 1994 (P.L. 103-322). The program has awarded funds to the Alzheimer's Association of America since FY1996 to protect and locate missing individuals with dementia through a patient identification program, as well as outreach and education efforts. In 2000, Congress passed Kristen's Act (P.L. 106-468) to permit the Department of Justice (DOJ) to make grants to establish a national clearinghouse for missing adults and provide technical assistance to law enforcement agencies in locating these individuals. From FY2002 through FY2006, DOJ made grants to the National Center for Missing Adults (NCMA) for these purposes. In addition, federal DNA Initiative has also supported efforts to recover missing persons and identify unidentified human remains by funding DNA analysis and providing technical assistance on using this analysis. Both DOJ and NCMA have established databases to collect and disseminate information to law enforcement on missing adults, their relatives, and unidentified human remains. These databases have overlapping but distinct features, and have limited capacity to share information.

Policymakers and other stakeholders have increasingly focused on two issues related to adults who go missing: whether to provide federal assistance to states and localities to develop alert systems and technology to locate missing adults; and possibly expanding federal involvement in cases of missing adults with diminished mental capacity. Another issue is the coordination of the databases on missing persons.

INTRODUCTION

Adults may go missing due to choice; an abduction or foul play; a physical or developmental disability; a natural catastrophe that displaces individuals, such as Hurricanes Katrina and Rita; or certain high-risk behaviors, including gang involvement or drug use, among other circumstances.

State and local laws govern how criminal justice entities respond to missing adult cases. This response is complicated by a number of factors. Unlike children, adults have the legal right to go missing in most cases and may do so to seek protection from a domestic abuser and other related reasons.[1] Further, law enforcement agencies may be hesitant to devote resources to missing adult cases, given competing priorities. Law enforcement agencies within and across states also respond differently to missing adult cases. Some states mandate that law enforcement officials take reports without a waiting period, while other states require at least a 24-hour waiting period after the person is believed to be missing.[2]

The federal government has not been involved in assisting state and local law enforcement entities with missing adult cases in the same way it has with missing children cases. Federal law requires law enforcement to report missing children and young adults under the age of 21 to the Federal Bureau of Investigation's (FBI) National Crime Information Center (NCIC), a federal database of crime and missing person information; reporting missing adults to the database is voluntary. In addition, since 1985, Congress has appropriated funding to the Missing and Exploited Children's Program to coordinate a federal response to missing children cases and to create and maintain a national clearinghouse that assists law enforcement and families with these cases.[3]

In recent years, the federal government has increasingly played a role in both (1) preventing certain types of missing adult incidents and (2) recovering adults who go missing, including those who are deceased and for whom only remains provide clues to their identity and circumstances surrounding their disappearance. In 1994, Congress authorized the Missing Alzheimer's Disease Patient Alert program under the Violent Crime Control and Law Enforcement Act of 1994 (P.L. 103-322) to assist in locating missing individuals with Alzheimer's disease and other forms of dementia through a patient identification program, as well as outreach and education efforts. In 2000, Congress authorized the Department of Justice (DOJ), through Kristen's Act (P.L. 106-468), to make grants to establish a national clearinghouse for missing adults and provide technical assistance to law enforcement agencies in locating missing adults. The federal government has also supported efforts to establish databases to track and identify missing adults, their relatives, and unidentified human remains. Some advocates of missing adults and policymakers have called for the federal government to expand its role in missing adult cases. For example, these advocates and policymakers would like the federal government to assist states by creating or expanding missing adult alert programs that serve as a warning to the public about cases of missing adults, much like the AMBER (America's Missing: Broadcast Emergency Response) Alert program for missing children.

The first section of this report discusses demographics and record keeping of missing adults and unidentified remains, and some of the factors that may contribute to the disappearance of adults. This section also discusses federally funded databases that are used to track data on missing adults and unidentified individuals. The second section of the report describes the federal programs and initiatives to assist in locating missing adults, including funding data where applicable. Finally, the third section discusses issues about the federal role in missing adult cases.

Why Do Adults Go Missing?

Certain circumstances can make adults vulnerable to going missing. Adults may go missing because of an abduction or foul play. A physical or developmental disability or cognitive disorder, such as Alzheimer's disease and other forms of dementia, may also contribute to a missing episode. Adults with dementia have been identified as high-risk for going missing by advocates for older adults. According to the Alzheimer's Association, as many as 5 million people in the U.S. suffer from Alzheimer's disease and related dementia, and about 60% of those will wander away from their homes or health care facilities.[4] Further, a natural catastrophe can displace individuals and make their whereabouts unknown to others. Approximately 13,000 adults were reported missing in the days following Hurricanes Katrina and Rita in 2005.[5] Finally, other adults vulnerable to missing incidents may include those with high-risk lifestyles, such as individuals who abuse drugs or are gang involved, and those that have a history of victimization, including domestic violence.[6]

Data on Missing Adults and Unidentified Decedents

There is no definitive estimate of the number of adults who go missing, because some adults are not known to be missing or are not reported to databases that compile data on missing persons. However, three federally supported data sources provide some insight into this number: the Missing Person File at the FBI's National Crime Information Center; the FBI's National DNA Index System (NDIS), which stores information on offenders and arrestees, forensic evidence, as well as individuals believed to be missing, their relatives, and unidentified human remains; and the National Missing and Unidentified Persons System (NamUs), administered by DOJ's National Institute of Justice (NIJ). The National Center for Missing Adults (NCMA), a clearinghouse in Glendale, AZ, that assists the families of missing adults and law enforcement agencies, also has a database on missing adults; NCMA was funded with a DOJ grant authorized by Kristen's Act from FY2002 through FY2006. Profiles of missing individuals entered into one database do not necessarily populate other databases, although some missing individuals may be reported to more than one of the databases. Therefore, numbers of missing persons should not be added across any of the databases.

The NCIC Unidentified Person File, NamUs, and NDIS contain information about unidentified decedents. However, the true number of unidentified missing adult cases is unknown because remains can go undiscovered, or if they are recovered, they may not be reported to the databases or retained. In a census conducted by DOJ in 2004, medical examiners and coroners reported a total of 13,486 unidentified human remains on record, though about 51% of medical examiner and coroners' offices lacked policies for retaining records such as x-rays, DNA, or fingerprints that could identify missing individuals.[7] (The report also found that 90% of offices serving large jurisdictions did retain such records.) Further, medical examiners and coroners estimated that about 4,400 unidentified human decedents were reported in an average year, with approximately 1,000 (23.0%) remaining unidentified after one year. Another DOJ study estimated, using death records reported to the Centers for Disease Control and Prevention from 1980 through 2004, that as many as 10,300 of these records were for unidentified decedents. This number is an approximation, as states do not uniformly specify on the death certificate when a person's identity is not known.[8] In addition, the criteria used by DOJ to search the death records may have included individuals whose identities were known, as well as unidentified individuals who were later identified.

The discussion below will show that the databases range in the number of profiles they contain, as well as the type of information they collect (e.g., basic demographic profiles, DNA profiles, etc.). *Note that only the data on missing persons and unidentified decedents, as reported in NCIC, are updated in this report.* The discussion also raises the question about whether these databases can, or should, share data or indicate that data about an individual profile is available in another database (some cross-referencing between the databases now occurs, though on a limited basis).

National Crime Information Center Missing Person and Unidentified Person Files

The NCIC within the FBI's Criminal Justice Information Services (CJIS) Division maintains statistics on missing adults and unidentified decedents.[9] The NCIC is a computerized index of documented information concerning crimes and criminals of nationwide interest and a locator file for missing and unidentified persons. Since October 1, 1975, the NCIC has maintained records of missing persons (known as the Missing Person File) who are reported to the FBI by federal, state, and local law enforcement agencies, foreign criminal justice agencies, and authorized courts. The Missing Person File was created in response to a request in 1974 from the NCIC Advisory Policy Board (APB).[10] The APB is composed of local, state, and federal criminal justice and national security agencies and advises the FBI on criminal justice information matters. The Missing Person File includes records for individuals who are missing because they

- have a proven physical or mental disability,
- are missing under circumstances indicating that they may be in physical danger,
- are missing under circumstances indicating their disappearance may not have been voluntary,
- are under the age of 21 and do not meet the above criteria,
- are missing after a catastrophe, or
- are 21 and older and do not meet any of the above criteria but for whom there is a reasonable concern for their safety.

These categories are presented in further detail in **Table A-1** in the **Appendix**. Pursuant to the National Child Search Assistance Act of 1990 (Title XXXVII of the Crime Control Act of 1990, P.L. 101-647), records of missing children under age 18 *must* be immediately entered into the Missing Person File. The act also requires the Attorney General to publish an annual statistical summary of the Missing Person File. Suzanne's Law, under the Prosecutorial Remedies and Other Tools to End the Exploitation of Children

Today Act of 2003 (PROTECT Act, P.L. 108-21), requires law enforcement to also immediately submit information about missing adults to the NCIC ages 18 through 20. Law enforcement agencies are not mandated under federal law to submit missing person records of adults over the age of 21 into the Missing Person File. Therefore, although records of missing adults are captured, the NCIC does not include the complete number of adults who go missing and are not reported to the database.

Missing Person Data for 2010[11]

As of January 1, 2011, there were 85,820 individual records (entered in 2010 and previous years) remaining in the Missing Person File. Of these, 47,315 (55.1%) were for missing adults ages 18 and older and 38,505 (44.9%) were for children ages 17 and younger.

In calendar year 2010, 692,944 individuals of all ages were reported missing to the NCIC. Also in that same year, approximately 703,316 missing person records were cleared or canceled; some of these records were entered prior to 2010. Of all individuals reported missing in 2010, a total of 161,016 (23.2%) were ages 18 and older. **Table A-1** in the **Appendix** summarizes the number of missing cases entered in 2008 through 2010 for individuals ages 18 and older under the six missing person categories listed above. The highest number of missing adults went missing for an unspecified reason, but there was a reasonable concern for their safety.

Of all adults ages 18 and older reported missing in 2010, most were male (58.4%). The majority (65.1%) of missing adults were white, followed by individuals who were black (28.1%), of an unknown race (2.9%), Asian (2.8%),[12] and American Indian or Alaskan Native (1.1%). African Americans appear to be overrepresented compared to their share of the general population by more than 10 percentage points.[13] The NCIC does not report on the Hispanic origin of missing individuals, and NCIC users are instructed to enter records for Hispanic individuals using the race code (American Indian or Alaskan Native, Asian or Pacific Islander, black, or white) that most closely represents that individual as perceived by the law enforcement official.[14]

Unidentified Missing Persons

Some individuals who go missing may be deceased, and their remains, intact or not, may be the only available clues concerning their identity and circumstances surrounding their disappearance. Since 1983, the NCIC has taken reports of unidentified missing persons, pursuant to the passage of the Missing Children Act of 1982 (P.L. 97-292). The act required the FBI to "acquire, collect, classify, and preserve any information which would assist in the identification of any deceased individual who has not been identified after the discovery of such deceased individual."[15] Pursuant to this requirement, reports are taken of unidentified deceased persons, persons of any age who are living and unable to determine their identity, and unidentified catastrophe victims. Reports may include information about bodies found shortly after death, when a person's remains may be fairly intact, as well as skeletal remains.

As of January 1, 2011, the Unidentified Remains File included 7,539 unidentified persons. Nearly all (7,390) of the entries were for deceased unidentified bodies; the remaining were for unidentified catastrophe victims and living persons who could not be identified, either because they could not identify themselves or refused to disclose their identity. The total number of unidentified persons in the NCIC may represent just a fraction of the true number of missing remains.

National DNA Index System[16]

Another federally funded database stores DNA records, including for missing adults and unidentified remains, and was authorized under the DNA Identification Act of 1994 as part the Violent Crime Control and Law Enforcement Act of 1994 (P.L. 103-322). This database is known as NDIS. P.L. 103-322 specified that the FBI could establish an index of DNA identification records of persons convicted of crimes, analyses of DNA samples recovered from crime scenes, and analyses from unidentified human remains.[17] A fourth category of records for relatives of missing persons was added in 1999 by the Consolidated Appropriations Act of 2000 (P.L. 106-113). DNA laboratories may enter DNA information into NDIS that involves one of the four categories of records, as well as the records of missing adults. The data are first entered by authorized users into the Local DNA Index System (LDIS), which can then populate the central laboratory for each state, known as a State DNA Index System (SDIS). Only SDIS laboratories may upload DNA profiles directly to the NDIS. LDIS or SDIS laboratories can conduct searches of their own databases prior to uploading the data to NDIS. Searches of data entered by other states into NDIS are conducted by the FBI Laboratory, which automatically searches new DNA data when profiles are submitted by the states.

NDIS contains over 6 million profiles in five databases: offenders and arrestees database, forensic evidence database, missing unidentified human remains database, missing person database, and biological relatives of missing persons database.[18] Most of the DNA profiles are those stored in the criminal and forensic evidence databases. The three missing person databases are part of the FBI Laboratory's National Missing Person DNA Database (NMPDD) program, which works to identify missing and unidentified persons based on available DNA profiles and other clues.[19] The unidentified human remains database contains DNA profiles from the remains of individuals that cannot be identified by fingerprint; dental, medical, or anthropological examinations; and of individuals who are living, but are unidentifiable using typical investigative methods (e.g., children and others who cannot or refuse to identify themselves). The relatives of missing persons database contains DNA profiles that are voluntarily submitted by the relatives of known missing individuals. Finally, the missing person database contains DNA records of missing persons obtained from their belongings or derived from the profiles of their relatives.

The three missing persons databases can be searched against one another. The Combined DNA Index System (CODIS) is the software in NDIS that compares various DNA profiles, and if a match is made between two sets of DNA profiles, the software sends an electronic message to the laboratories that contributed the samples. DNA analysts at the laboratories review the data to confirm the match. The laboratories are responsible for alerting the investigating law enforcement agency, medical examiner, coroner, or medical-legal authority of the results. The FBI is continuing to develop technology, including software to conduct kinship DNA analyses, and is using meta-data (e.g., sex, date of last sighting, and age), that is intended to assist in locating missing persons.[20]

The National Missing and Unidentified Persons System[21]

NamUs was established in July 2007 as an online repository for information about missing persons and unidentified remains.[22] The system was created as part of the President's DNA Initiative,[23] described below, out of concern that state and local law enforcement agencies, medical examiners, and coroners are not required to report missing adult and unidentified decedent cases to the NCIC, and therefore, the true number of missing adults is unknown.[24] To further investigate this issue, DOJ appointed an expert panel of medical examiners and coroners, which ultimately confirmed the need for a central reporting system for unidentified human remains. These efforts also led DOJ to establish and fund NamUs. NamUs is composed of two databases, one for missing persons and the other for unidentified remains.

The Missing Person Database serves as a repository for information on missing persons that can be entered by law enforcement agencies or members of the public. Profiles of missing individuals may include photographs and information about the circumstances around their disappearance, their dental records, DNA, physical appearance, and police contact information, among other items. Users of the website—members of the public, law enforcement, coroners, and medical examiners—may search the database based on these attributes. The database also includes information about state statutes on recovering missing persons as well as links to state missing person clearinghouses, which are maintained by state law enforcement agencies or advocacy organizations and provide information about missing adults.

The Unidentified Remains Database is available for medical examiners and coroners to upload their cases.[25] Website users may view profiles of the unidentified remains; however, only law enforcement agencies and other authorized entities may enter information and review additional information and photographs that are not available to the public. Some of the profiles are fully intact, whereas others include pieces of the missing person's body or information about the remains and where they were found. Website users can also search based on characteristics such as demographics, anthropologic analysis, the NCIC record number, dental information, and distinct body features.

During the development of NamUs, representatives from NDIS, NCIC, the Violent Criminal Apprehension Program (ViCAP), described below, and Integrated Automated Fingerprint Identification System (IAFIS), described below, were involved as partners in working groups and focus groups that developed requirements for the system.[26] Also, according to DOJ, state and local practitioners participated in developing the requirements of the system and made recommendations for specific technology upgrades that were incorporated.

OTHER DATABASES THAT CAN STORE INFORMATION ABOUT MISSING PERSONS

Integrated Automated Fingerprint Identification System (IAFIS): IAFIS is an electronic database that stores information on fingerprints and corresponding criminal histories. This information is submitted voluntarily by state, local, and federal law enforcement agencies. The database includes more than 55 million subjects in its Criminal Master File; nearly 50 records are for missing persons. Law enforcement agencies that submit electronic fingerprints receive electronic responses to criminal 10-print fingerprint submissions within two hours and within 24 hours for civil fingerprint submissions (i.e., background checks for employment and other non-criminal justice related purposes). The response indicates whether an individual has a criminal history. IAFIS is administered by the FBI's Criminal Justice Information Services Division. For additional information, see http://www.fbi.gov/hq/cjisd/iafis.htm.

Violent Criminal Apprehension Program (ViCAP): ViCAP is a data center that collects and analyzes information on crimes, including missing person cases where the circumstances indicate a strong possibility of foul play and the victim is still missing. However, few missing adult cases are actually entered because, according to the FBI, the NCIC does not automatically populate the ViCAP database. Cases with an arrested or identified offender can be entered into the ViCAP system by law enforcement investigators for database comparison and possible matching with unsolved cases. Once a case is entered into the ViCAP database, it is compared continuously against all other entries on the basis of certain aspects of the crime. The purpose of this process is to detect signature aspects and traits of the crime to allow ViCAP personnel with the FBI's Criminal Justice Information Services Division to identify crimes that have been committed by the same offender. For additional information, see http://www.fbi.gov/hq/isd/ ciirg/ncavc.htm#vicap.

National Center for Missing Adults (NCMA)/Let's Bring Them Home: NCMA, which merged in 2009 with Let's Bring Them Home, a non-profit organization, has received funding from DOJ for its efforts to work on behalf of missing adults and their families. NCMA maintains a database of the number of adults who are reported missing to the organization by family members or law enforcement. Since the database began operating in 2003, NCMA has received more than 25,000 reports of missing person ages 18 and older. About one-third of the cases are pending. The database classifies characteristics of the missing persons, such as disabilities, history of domestic violence, homelessness, missing from group homes, and other categories. About half of missing persons that have been recorded in the database have a diagnosed mental condition that requires care or medication; approximately one-third have a mental illness or diminished mental capacity; and the remaining share have Alzheimer's disease or related dementia, alcohol or chemical dependency, or another unspecified disability.

Source: Congressional Research Service.

Comparison and Interaction of Databases

Table A-2 in the **Appendix** summarizes some of the features of the databases on missing persons and unidentified remains, as well as the entities that may access them. As described above, NDIS includes DNA profiles and IAFIS includes fingerprint records, whereas some of the other databases only indicate whether these records are available. These other databases also tend to include more general information about missing persons and the circumstances surrounding their disappearance. Further, IAFIS and ViCAP have a broader mandate to store criminal justice-related data and do not focus, per se, on missing adult cases. The databases are not linked and do not populate one another.[27] This has been identified as a concern of DOJ's National Missing Persons Taskforce, discussed below.

Records are submitted to most of the databases by authorized law enforcement agencies, state missing persons clearinghouses, medical examiners and coroners, or DNA laboratories. Nearly all of the databases can be accessed exclusively by the federal government or authorized law enforcement and other personnel; however, records in NamUs and the NCMA database can also be reviewed by the public, though sometimes only on a limited basis for NamUs. All of the databases, except the one administered by NCMA, are overseen by the federal government. Further, federal funds have been used to develop, expand, and/or administer each of the databases.

Federal Role in Recovering Missing Adults

Efforts to recover missing adults are primarily under the jurisdiction of state and local governments. These efforts may be complicated by a number of factors. Unlike children, adults have the legal right to go missing in most cases and can do so to seek protection from a domestic abuser and other reasons.[28] Further, law enforcement agencies may be hesitant to devote resources to missing adult cases given competing priorities. In addition, law enforcement agencies within and across states respond differently to missing adult cases. Some states mandate that law enforcement officials take reports without a waiting period, whereas other states require at least a 24-hour waiting period after the person is believed to be missing.[29]

In recent years, the federal government has increasingly played a role both in preventing certain types of missing adult incidents and in working to recover adults who go missing, including those who are deceased and for whom only remains provide clues to the circumstances surrounding their disappearance. In addition to funding or operating databases that track information about missing adults and unidentified remains, the federal government has undertaken other related efforts, including support for (1) the DNA Initiative, created under President George W. Bush, which has focused on identifying the remains of unidentified deceased individuals; (2) National Missing Persons Task Force, with its emphasis on achieving greater cooperation among the various federal databases; (3) the Missing Alzheimer's Disease Patient Alert program to prevent missing episodes and locate missing individuals with Alzheimer's disease and related dementia; (4) activities funded under Kristen's Act to locate missing adults; and (5) the National Center for Missing and Exploited Children (NCMEC), which works to recover missing children and adults ages 18 to 21 who are reported to the agency as missing by law enforcement officials. The Missing Alzheimer's Disease Patient Alert program and activities funded under Kristen's Act have specifically received congressional appropriations for missing adult activities. The other activities have been funded under appropriations for initiatives or programs that encompass more than missing adult activities.

DNA Initiative and Related Activities

In March 2003, President Bush announced a new DNA Initiative to promote the use of forensic DNA technology to solve crimes, protect individuals from wrongful prosecution, and identify missing persons.[30] Within the past several years, Congress has appropriated funding to DOJ to carry out the following activities to assist with locating missing adults and unidentified remains:[31]

- sample analysis of unidentified human remains and family reference samples;[32]
- standardized sample DNA collection kits for unidentified remains of missing persons;
- evaluation and implementation of advanced DNA technologies to facilitate the analysis of skeletal remains;
- focus group on using DNA technology to assist the identification of human remains;
- training and technical assistance on using DNA to identify missing persons and unidentified remains (see below);

- census of medical examiners and coroners and inventory of unidentified remains; and
- NamUs Unidentified Decedent Database.

Also as part of the DNA Initiative, DOJ held two regional missing person forums and the First National Strategy Meeting on Identifying the Missing in 2005.[33] (No other national meetings have been held to date.) The forums provided attendees, including medical examiners, coroners, law enforcement personnel, managers of state missing children clearinghouses, family members of missing persons, forensic scientists, and policymakers, with information about resources to solve missing person and unidentified human remains cases in their jurisdictions. The forums addressed topics including model state programs for recovering missing persons and unidentified remains, reference sample DNA collection kits, and evidence repositories. The national strategy meeting was convened with the same groups of attendees described above to identify policies and practices, including the use of DNA, to solve missing person and unidentified decedent cases. The Task Force also created model state legislation to encourage states to adopt laws that improve the ability of law enforcement to locate and return missing persons, identify human remains, and provide timely information to family members of missing persons.[34]

National Missing Person's Taskforce[35]

As part of the DNA Initiative, in 2005, NIJ and FBI were directed by DOJ leadership to establish a national task force to assess how to better encourage, facilitate, and achieve greater use of federal missing person databases to solve missing persons cases and identify human remains. In response to this directive, NIJ and the FBI convened the National Missing Persons Taskforce, composed of a broad cross-section of criminal justice officials, forensic science experts, and victim advocates. The task force met July 2005 through January 2006 to address, among other issues, the federal databases that store information on missing persons and unidentified human remains. According to DOJ, members of the task force convened these meetings to better understand and improve the information sharing tools and DNA technologies available to solve cases involving missing persons and unidentified decedents.

Missing Alzheimer's Disease Patient Alert Program[36]

The Violent Crime Control and Law Enforcement Act of 1994 (P.L. 103-322) authorized the Missing Alzheimer's Disease Patient Alert program to provide grants to locally based organizations to protect and locate missing patients with Alzheimer's disease and related dementia. Funding was authorized at $900,000 for each of FY1996, FY1997, and FY1998. Congress has appropriated funding for the program from FY1996 through FY2010. Funding more than doubled from FY2008 to FY2009.

Table 1. Appropriations for Missing Alzheimer's Disease Patient Alert Program, FY2002 through FY2011, and Funding Proposed by the Obama Administration for FY2012 ($ in Millions)

FY2002	FY2003	FY2004	FY2005	FY2006	FY2007	FY2008	FY2009	FY2010	FY2011	FY2012 Request
$0.90	$0.86	$0.85	$0.87	$0.84	$0.84	$0.94	$2.0	$2.0	$2.0	0

Sources: FY2000 from H.Rept. 106-680; FY2001 from H.Rept. 107-139; FY2002 from H.Rept. 107-278; FY2003 from H.Rept. 108-10; FY2004 from H.Rept. 108-401; FY2005 from H.Rept. 108-792; FY2006 from H.Rept. 109-272. FY2007 appropriation is based on FY2006 enacted minus a 1.28% rescission, as per P.L. 110-5. FY2008 from U.S. House, Committee on Rules, Joint Explanatory Statement to Accompany FY2008 Consolidated Appropriations Amendment to H.R. 2764 (P.L. 110-161), Division B. FY2009 from U.S. House, Committee on Rules, Joint Explanatory Statement to Accompany FY2009 Consolidated Appropriations Amendment to H.R. 1105 (P.L. 111-8), Division B. FY2010 from U.S. House, Committee on Rules, Conference Report to Accompany Consolidated Appropriations Act, 2010 (P.L. 111-117), Division B. FY2011 appropriation is based on Department of Defense and Full-Year Continuing Appropriations Act, 2011 (P.L. 112-10), minus a 0.2% rescission from FY2010, or $1,960,000. FY2012 from U.S. Department of Justice, *Office of Justice Programs, FY2012 Performance Budget*, p. 250.

These funds, administered by DOJ's Office of Justice Programs, have been awarded to the Alzheimer's Association of America. Table 1 shows funding for the program from FY2002 through FY2011 and the FY2012 proposal to cut the program.

Safe Return Program[37]

DOJ has awarded funds through the Missing Alzheimer's Disease Patient Alert program to the Alzheimer's Association of America in each year since FY1996. These funds have been used to establish and carry out the Safe

Return Program, which works to protect and locate missing individuals with Alzheimer's and related dementia. Wandering may pose a significant, if not life threatening, danger to the personal health, safety, and welfare of those with dementia.[38] This may occur from exposure to the elements; lack of food; dehydration or lack of medication for extended periods of time; and general inability to think, act, or communicate in a way that could assist them. Nevertheless, it is not uncommon for persons with dementia to wander from their homes, sometimes repeatedly. The Alzheimer's Association reports that six out of 10 people with Alzheimer's disease will wander during the course of the disease.

The Safe Return program provides enrollees with a bracelet indicating that the individual is memory impaired and includes a toll-free, 24-hour emergency response number to call if the person is found wandering or lost. The call is routed to the nearest local chapter of the organization, which works to reunite the person with his or her caregiver, including long-term care facilities. The local chapter obtains information—through the organization's central database that includes personal and medical information and sometimes a picture of the enrollee—about the individual, and then contacts the caregiver or local law enforcement agency. Family members or caregivers with a loved one or care recipient enrolled in the program may also contact the Alzheimer's Association in the event that he or she goes missing.

The Alzheimer's Association reports that in two thirds of cases, the enrolled missing individual and caretaker are immediately reunited. In the one-third of cases that are truly missing persons incidents, local law enforcement agencies are involved, and the local chapter provides assistance during search and rescue efforts. The chapter also provides emotional support to the family and can serve as a media contact. In addition to these services, the Alzheimer's Association works with families to identify needed resources to prevent missing incidents and support the caregivers of individuals with Alzheimer's and dementia.

Approximately 120,000 individuals are enrolled in the Safe Return program.[39] The program reportedly has helped in the safe return of over 8,000 people since 1993. The organization also provides training materials to law enforcement agencies about individuals with Alzheimer's, and how to recognize wandering behavior or individuals with dementia who are engaging in unsafe or uncharacteristic behavior, such as driving or shoplifting. Some chapters have partnerships with local law enforcement agencies to educate them about wandering behavior, but the level of contact varies across the country. Most chapters coordinate with state units on aging to make them aware of the organization and Safe Return program.

Kristen's Act

In 2000, Congress passed Kristen's Act (P.L. 106-468), named after Kristen Modafferi, who has been missing since 1997. Kristen was 18 when she disappeared and her family was unable to access services through the National Center for Missing and Exploited Children because, at the time, the organization only provided assistance to missing incident cases for children under age 18. NCMEC now provides services for missing young adults ages 18 to 21, pursuant to Suzanne's Law, which requires law enforcement to also immediately submit information about missing adults to the NCIC ages 18 through 20. Kristen's Act authorized $1 million in funding for each of FY2001 to FY2004 and permitted the Attorney General to make grants to assist law enforcement agencies in locating missing adults; maintain a database for tracking adults believed by law enforcement to be endangered due to age, diminished mental capacity, and possible foul play; maintain statistical information on missing adults; provide resources and referrals to the families of missing adults; and establish and maintain a national clearinghouse for missing adults.

Kristen's Act grants were made from FY2002 through FY2006 through the Edward Byrne Discretionary Grant Program to NCMA, though funding authorization expired at the end of FY2004. Funding levels ranged from $150,000 to $1.7 million. Kristen's Act grants have not been funded since FY2006.

Overview of Services Provided by the National Center for Missing Adults[40]

NCMA began in 1995 as the missing adult division of the Nation's Missing Children Organization. NCMA received funding under Kristen's Act to expand its efforts to recover missing adults beginning in FY2002 and received this funding through FY2006. Although the organization has operated since this time, it does so on a more limited scale. It currently receives funding from local governments and private organizations. In 2009, NCMA merged with Let's Bring Them Home, a non-profit organization that provides education and resources on missing persons. According to NCMA, this partnership is providing financial stability to the organization.[41]

NCMA is not an investigating agency and only accepts missing adult cases that have first been reported to a law enforcement agency. A missing adult case can be registered with NCMA by a law enforcement official or family member (or significant other, friend, and certain other individuals) of the missing individual. The reporting parties complete a registration form that requests any available descriptive information, circumstances of disappearance, law enforcement case number, NCIC number, investigating law enforcement agency contact information, and other information. The reporting party may also submit a photo.

A case manager is assigned to the missing person case and will enter any relevant information, including answers from the registration form, types of services provided, and dates and summaries of all conversations with the reporting party, among other information. The case manager contacts the law enforcement agency to verify case information and that the missing person has been entered into the NCIC Missing Person File. (If the law enforcement agency does not enter the record into the NCIC, the case manager will offer to assist with referrals and resources.) The case manager then determines which services will be provided by the organization and contacts the family to let them know about these services. NCMA may also add the missing person's profile and picture to its website (www.missingadults.org), send missing person flyers to the family and law enforcement, assist with press releases, help generate or manage media attention, and maintain routine contact with the family.

National Center for Missing and Exploited Children

The National Center for Missing and Exploited Children is a primary component of the federally funded Missing and Exploited Children's Program.[42] Although NCMEC's mission is to recover missing children under age 18, it also provides services for missing young adults ages 18 through 20, pursuant to Suzanne's Law, which requires law enforcement to also immediately submit information about missing adults to the NCIC ages 18 through 20. This law changed the upper age limit of individuals who must be entered into the NCIC.

NCMEC processes young adult cases differently than cases for missing children.[43] NCMEC will accept a young adult case only if it is reported by a law enforcement entity—and not by parents, spouses, partners, or others—because the organization relies on law enforcement personnel to verify that the young adult is missing due to foul play or other reasons that would cause concern about the individual's whereabouts, such as diminished mental capacity. NCMEC then assists in recovery efforts for these adults as it would for children under age 18. A case manager in the Missing Children's Division is assigned to serve as the single point of contact for the searching family and to provide technical assistance to locate abductors and recover missing children and young adults.

ISSUES

The various federal data systems to record information about missing adults raise the question about the need and ability for the systems to share this information. Further, federal and state policymakers and other stakeholders have increasingly focused on three issues related to adults who go missing: (1) coordinating databases on missing persons; (2) assisting states with building the capacity to develop both alert systems to inform the public about missing older adults and technology to recover these individuals; and (3) extending federal protections to missing adults with diminished mental capacity. Where applicable, this section discusses pending legislation that would address these issues.

Coordination of Federally Funded Databases on Missing Persons and Unidentified Decedents

The first section of this report discussed the various federally funded databases that store information on missing persons and unidentified decedents. These databases do not currently populate one another, although some of the databases indicate whether information about a particular individual is available in another database. This limitation raises the question about whether the federal government can and should develop technology to enable the databases to coordinate, although concerns about privacy and funding would likely need to be addressed. DOJ appears to have begun initial discussions about the interactions of the databases through its Missing Person Task Force. Further, the NamUs database could ultimately serve as a central repository on missing adults and unidentified remains.

Alert Systems

Silver or Senior Alerts[44]

Alert systems, known as Silver or Senior Alerts, have been established in multiple states.[45] These alert systems were created out of concern for the safety of seniors and other at-risk adult populations who are prone to wandering due to a physical or cognitive disability or medical condition such as Alzheimer's or other forms of dementia. Some missing adult alert programs are modeled after the states' AMBER Alert system for abducted children.[46]

Issuing alerts to law enforcement agencies and the public for missing vulnerable adults in some of the states appears to be at the discretion of the law enforcement agency—local or state or both—and is not required of the agency.[47] In addition, state alert systems vary in terms of the target population for issuing an alert (i.e., older adults with dementia versus any adult with a disability). Most law enforcement agencies have the ability to disseminate the alert to law enforcement agencies and media in the local area, region, statewide, and other states. For example, the Texas Division of Emergency Management disseminates information within the alert advisory area to local, state, and federal law enforcement agencies, primary media outlets, the Texas Department of Transportation, the Texas Lottery Commission, and the Independent Bankers Association of Texas.

Some advocates have raised concerns that alert systems may not be useful for some adults who go missing. For example, it is reported that nearly all (94%) persons with Alzheimer's disease who wander are found less than 1.5 miles from home and almost 30% are found among makeshift shelters under brush or briar.[48] Further, there is concern that alerting the media repeatedly about a missing adult case could desensitize the public to the issue of wandering. Some advocates suggest that policymakers may wish to consider Silver Alerts in combination with a combination of other policy approaches.[49]

Tracking Technology[50]

Electronic monitoring services for individuals who are susceptible to going missing are being implemented by some state and local law enforcement agencies with technology developed by Project Lifesaver International, a nonprofit organization that administers the Project Lifesaver program. Project Lifesaver uses a personalized wristband that emits a signal to track individuals prone to going missing. The wristband is worn by the clients continuously, and each month, a law enforcement officer or trained volunteer visits with the clients to replace the wristband batteries and provide referrals to clients and their caregivers in need of social services. When family members or caregivers report to the designated Project Lifesaver agency—typically a local law enforcement or first responder agency—that the client is missing, a search and rescue team responds to the wanderer's area to search using a mobile locator tracking system.

Project Lifesaver grew out of local law enforcement experience with search and rescue efforts for missing persons with Alzheimer's and other forms of dementia. The target population of the program has expanded to include children with special needs such as autism and Down's syndrome and to anyone else that may be at risk of wandering for a medical reason. In addition to providing the technology, the program trains the designated agency to communicate with persons with Alzheimer's disease and other disorders.

Project Lifesaver International reported that the tracking technology is used by hundreds of law enforcement agencies in most states and in some parts of Canada. According to Project Lifesaver International, the benefits from the program include saving law enforcement and search and rescue response time and resources in locating missing persons due to wandering. The organization reports that search times have been reduced from hours and days for searches without radio technology to minutes in searches that use the technology. In over 1,500 searches, there have been no reported serious injuries or deaths and recovery times have averaged less than 30 minutes.[51]

SPECIAL FEDERAL PROTECTIONS FOR VULNERABLE MISSING ADULTS

There is currently no federal mandate to locate missing adults who function cognitively as children. A bill in the 110th Congress, the Audrey Nerenberg Act (H.R. 271), sought to extend the same federal assistance to these adults that is provided for missing children. The legislation proposed to change the definition of "missing child" under the Missing Children's Assistance Act, as amended, to include individuals determined to have a mental capacity of less than 18 years of age as determined by an appropriate medical authority. The act did not specify which adults with a diminished mental capacity would be protected. For example, the legislation could have included disorders as diverse as Down's syndrome and Alzheimer's, and if left for states to decide, the definition could have varied widely from one state to another. The bill also did not define the rights of adults with cognitive disabilities who want to go missing and may choose to do so for legitimate reasons.

H.R. 271 would have essentially required the National Center for Missing and Exploited Children—which receives most of the funding from the federal Missing and Exploited Children's program, authorized by the Missing Children's Assistance Act—to work to recover any missing adults deemed eligible under H.R. 271. In response to the possibility that NCMEC would need to focus its work on certain vulnerable adults ages 21 and older, the organization has said that it would prefer to initially take on missing adults cases on a pilot basis to assess the issues and problems that may arise, such as varying state law definitions of diminished capacity.[52] According to NCMEC, "We would only take diminished capacity cases if requested to do so by a law enforcement agency. And given that these are cases of missing adults, who are not like children whose disappearance is presumed to be involuntary, we would likely need limited civil and criminal liability to prevent costly and burdensome lawsuits."

APPENDIX

Table A-1. National Crime Information Center (NCIC): Missing Entries of Adults Ages 18 and Older, 2008-2010

Category (as defined under the NCIC Operating Manual)	Number of Missing Adults and Share of Total Missing Adult Cases (2008)	Number of Missing Adults and Share of Total Missing Adult Cases (2009)	Number of Missing Adults and Share of Total Missing Adult Cases (2010)[a]
Disability: a person of any age who is missing and under proven mental/physical disability or senile, thereby subjecting himself/herself or others to personal and immediate danger.[b]	28,950 (17.7%)	28,824 (17.9%)	27,009 (16.8%)
Endangered: a person of any age who is missing under circumstances indicating that his/her physical safety may be in danger.	74,451 (45.6%)	71,070 (44.1%)	50,951 (31.6%)
Involuntary: a person of any age who is missing under circumstances indicating that the disappearance may not have been voluntary, i.e., abduction or kidnapping.	14,468 (8.9%)	14,290 (8.9%)	14,555 (9.0%)

Category (as defined under the NCIC Operating Manual)	Number of Missing Adults and Share of Total Missing Adult Cases (2008)	Number of Missing Adults and Share of Total Missing Adult Cases (2009)	Number of Missing Adults and Share of Total Missing Adult Cases (2010)[a]
Juvenile: a person under age 21 who is missing and does not meet any of the enter criteria set forth under the Disability, Endangered, Involuntary, or Catastrophe categories.	9,032 (5.5%)	7,658 (4.8%)	5,324 (3.3%)
Catastrophe: a person of any age who missing after a catastrophe.[b]	295 (0.2%)	267 (0.2%)	238 (0.2%)
Other: a person age 21 and older who does not meet any of the above criteria but for whom there is a reasonable concern for their safety; or a person who is under age 21 who is declared emancipated by the laws of his or her state of residence.	36,043 (22.1%)	38,956 (24.2%)	62,939 (39.1%)
Total	**163,239**	**161,065**	**161,016**

Source: Congressional Research Service presentation of data provided by the U.S. Department of Justice, Federal Bureau of Investigation, Criminal Justice Information Services Division on April 5, 2009; January 27, 2010; and January 18-19, 2011.

a. From 2009 to 2010, the share of missing adults who were reported in the "endangered" category decreased while the share of missing adults who were reported in the "other" category increased. According to the FBI, this is due to the change in the definition of the "other" category in August 2009. The definition changed from "a person age 18 or older not meeting the criteria for entry in any other category who is missing and for who there is a reasonable concern for his/her safety" to "a person age 21 and older not meeting the criteria for entry in any other category who is missing and for whom there is a reasonable concern for his/her safety or a person who is under 21 and declared emancipated by laws of his/her state of residence." This information was provided to the Congressional Research Service by the U.S. Department of Justice, Federal Bureau of Investigation, Criminal Justice Information Services Division on January 19, 2011.

b. According to the FBI, "proven physical or mental disability" refers to an individual who could have suicidal tendencies or a drug addiction, is a hemophiliac or diabetic, or has previously escaped custody, among other possible characteristics. A "catastrophe" refers to a disaster, such as an airplane crash, terrorist attack, natural disaster, among other possible scenarios. This information was provided to the Congressional Research Service by the U.S. Department of Justice, Federal Bureau of Investigation, Criminal Justice Information Services Division on December 26, 2007.

Table A-2. Databases of Missing Adults and Unidentified Remains

Database—Administering Agency or Organization	Features	Access to Database
National Crime Information Center (NCIC) Missing Person File and Unidentified Persons File—DOJ/FBI	The database includes descriptive information about the missing individual or their remains. Individuals are classified under one of six missing person categories or one of three unidentified missing person categories. The databases indicate whether DNA and fingerprinting information are available.	Data are reported by, and available to, authorized federal, state, and local criminal justice and non-criminal justice agencies.
National DNA Index System (NDIS)—DOJ/FBI	The system includes three databases for the DNA of missing persons, unidentified remains, and relatives of missing persons.	Data are reported by state and local DNA laboratories, in cooperation with state and local law enforcement officials. All profiles can be accessed by the FBI; some profiles can be accessed by the state and local DNA laboratories.
National Missing and Unidentified Persons System (NamUs)—DOJ/NIJ	The system is under construction and will include two databases for descriptive information and pictures about missing persons and unidentified remains. The unidentified remains database is operational, and features information about the location of the remains, distinguishing features, and law enforce-ment contact information, and whether DNA and dental records are available. The two databases will ultimately be linked.	Data are reported by, and available to, authorized federal, state, and local criminal justice and non-criminal justice agencies. Profiles can be accessed by these entities and the public, although the public may not have access to information and photographs for some profiles.

Database—Administering Agency or Organization	Features	Access to Database
National Center for Missing Adults (NCMA) Database—NCMA	The system includes descriptive information about missing adults, including information about the circumstances of the individual's disappearance, distingui-shing features, whether DNA and dental records are available, and law enforcement contact information, among other information.	Data are entered by NCMA staff after confirming that a missing adult report was first submitted to a law enforcement entity. Profiles can be access by the public.
Integrated Automated Fingerprint Identification System (IAFIS) — DOJ/FBI	The system includes fingerprints and corresponding criminal histories.	Data are reported by authorized international, federal, state, and local criminal justice and non-criminal justice agencies.
Violent Criminal Apprehension Program (ViCAP)—DOJ/FBI	The system includes information on crimes, including missing person cases where the circumstances indicate a strong possibility of foul play and the victim is still missing. The database entries are continuously compared on the basis of certain aspects of the crime.	Data are reported by authorized federal, state, and local criminal justice and non-criminal justice agencies.

Source: Congressional Research Service.

End Notes

[1] Guardians and the court system may limit the autonomy of some adults through conservatorship or guardianship arrangements.

[2] For differences among some states regarding waiting periods for taking reports, see http://www.find-the-missing.org/ states/index.htm.

[3] For further information, see CRS Report RL34050, *Missing and Exploited Children: Background, Policies, and Issues*, by Adrienne L. Fernandes-Alcantara.

[4] Ashlen Anderson, *Issue Kit: Public Policy Responses to Wandering Behavior*," Alzheimer's Association of America, September 2006. (Hereafter referenced Ashlen Anderson, *Public Policy Responses to Wandering Behavior*.) For a discussion of the incidence and prevalence of Alzheimer's disease, see CRS Report RL32970, *Biomedical Advances in Alzheimer's Disease*, by Michele M. Schoonmaker and Laura B. Shrestha.

[5] This information was provided to the Congressional Research Service by the National Center for Missing Adults on May 1, 2008.

[6] These groups have been identified as vulnerable to going missing by the National Center for Missing Adults.

[7] Matthew J. Hickman et al., *Medical Examiners and Coroners' Offices, 2004*, U.S. Department of Justice, Bureau of Justice Statistics, June 2007, at http://bjs.ojp.usdoj.gov/ content/pub/pdf/meco04.pdf.

[8] Kristen Hughes, *Unidentified Human Remains in the United States, 1980-2004*, U.S. Department of Justice, Bureau of Justice Statistics, November 2007, at *http://bjs.ojp.* usdoj.gov/ content/pub/pdf/uhrus04.pdf.

[9] Unless otherwise noted, this information was provided to the Congressional Research Service by the U.S. Department of Justice, Federal Bureau of Investigation, Criminal Justice Information Services Division on January 25, 2008. For further information about the current NCIC Advisory Policy Board, see http://www.fbi.gov/about-us/cjis/advisory-policy-board. The FBI is authorized to maintain the NCIC under 28 U.S.C. 434.

[10] The Missing Children Act of 1982 affirmed the need for the Missing Person File by requiring the FBI to "acquire, collect, classify, and preserve any information which would assist in the location of any missing person (including an unemancipated person as defined by the laws of the places of residence of such person) and provide confirmation as to any entry for such a person to the parent, legal guardian, or next of kin of that person." 28 U.S.C. 534(a). The FBI amended NCIC entry procedures in May 1999 to replace the phrase "unemancipated person" with "a person who is missing under the age of 18."

[11] Unless otherwise noted, this information was provided to the Congressional Research Service by the U.S. Department of Justice, Federal Bureau of Investigation, Criminal Justice Information Services Division on January 18, 2011.

[12] This includes individuals who identify as Native Hawaiian or Other Pacific Islander.

[13] For information about demographics of the general population, see *2005-2009 American Community Survey 5-year Estimates*, http://factfinder.census.gov/servlet/DatasetMainPage Servlet?_program=ACS&_submenuId=&_lang=en&_ts=.

[14] In October 1997, the Office of Management and Budget published revised standards for the reporting by federal agencies of statistics on race and ethnicity. The standards specify the racial categories of American Indian or Alaska Native, black or African American, Native Hawaiian or Other Pacific Islander, and white; and ethnic categories of Hispanic or Latino and Not Hispanic or Latino. However, the FBI received an exemption from this reporting requirement for the NCIC. According to the FBI, states are not required to comply with the racial and ethnic classifications, due to the uniqueness of crime data and the fact that the data are reported by state and local jurisdictions. This information was provided to the Congressional Research Service by the U.S. Department of Justice, Federal Bureau of Investigation, Criminal Justice Information Services Division on May 6, 2008.

[15] 28 U.S.C. 534(a).

[16] Unless otherwise noted, this information was provided to the Congressional Research Service by the U.S. Department of Justice, Federal Bureau of Investigation, Office of Congressional Affairs on June 18, 2008, and July 16, 2008.

[17] According to the FBI, the authority to include DNA from missing persons is derived from P.L. 103-322, because in order to identify unidentified remains, a search of missing person records must be conducted that compares those records to the records for unidentified remains. This information was provided to the Congressional Research Service by the Department of Justice, Federal Bureau of Investigation, Office of Congressional Affairs on August 8, 2008.

[18] The other two databases, the convicted offender database and forensic database, can be searched against one another to assist law enforcement personnel in solving crimes.

[19] In addition to conducting DNA analysis, the FBI Laboratory also assists state and local law enforcement agencies with investigations of missing persons involving examinations of

anthropology, trace evidence, facial reconstruction, fingerprinting, and toolmarking. These services are provided at no cost.

[20] U.S. Department of Justice, Federal Bureau of Investigation, "CODIS: Combined DNA Index System," at *http://www.fbi.gov/about-us/lab/codis*.

[21] Unless otherwise noted, this information is provided by U.S. Department of Justice, "About Missing Persons Database," NamUs, at http://www.namus.gov/index.htm.

[22] According to the Department of Justice, there is no specific statutory authority for NamUs; however, the agency derives its authority to establish the database from statutes on the general authorities of the National Institute of Justice (NIJ, 42 U.S.C. 3721-3723), which manages the database, to support research and develop tools and technologies, as well as statutes concerning the general authorities of NIJ's Office of Science and Technology (6 U.S.C. 161-165). This information was provided to the Congressional Research Service by the U.S. Department of Justice, Office of Justice Programs on June 16, 2008.

[23] The President's DNA Initiative was created under President George W. Bush.

[24] U.S. Department of Justice, "About Missing Persons Database," NamUs, at http://www.namus.gov/ index.htm.

[25] The database was initially developed in 2005 and 2006 as a public service project by the National Association of Medical Examiners, Occupational Research and Assessment, Inc. (ORAINC), and the International Association of Coroners and Medical Examiners.

[26] This information was provided to the Congressional Research Service by the U.S. Department of Justice, Office of Justice Programs on June 16, 2008.

[27] This may be due, in part, to concerns with protecting the privacy of individuals registered in the databases. For example, the DNA Identification Act of 1994 (P.L. 103-322) limit the accessibility of the profiles in NDIS for certain purposes.

[28] Guardians and the court system may limit the autonomy of some adults through conservatorship or guardianship arrangements.

[29] For differences among some states regarding waiting periods for taking reports, see http://www.find-the-missing.org/ states/index.htm.

[30] For additional information about the DNA Initiative, see CRS Report RL33489, *An Overview and Funding History of Select Department of Justice (DOJ) Grant Programs*, by Nathan James.

[31] The Justice for All Act of 2004 (P.L. 108-405) authorized funding for DNA technology to meet some of the activities set forth in the President's DNA Initiative. Sec. 308 of the act provides that the Attorney General may use DNA technology to identify missing persons and unidentified human remains. Sec. 308 further requires that each state or unit of local government that receives funding under the section is required to submit the DNA profiles of missing persons and unidentified human remains to the NDIS national missing persons database. According to the Department of Justice, no specific appropriation has been made pursuant to this section of the act.

[32] Laboratories that participate in NDIS conduct these sample analyses, and the DNA results are forwarded to the relevant missing person indexes in NDIS.

[33] For additional information, see The DNA Initiative, at http://www.dna.gov/.

[34] The model state legislation is at http://www.ncjrs.gov/pdffiles1/nij/210740v2.pdf.

[35] This information was provided to the Congressional Research Service by the U.S. Department of Justice, Office of Justice Programs on June 16, 2008.

[36] This section was co-authored with Kirsten J. Colello, Analyst in Gerontology.

[37] Unless otherwise noted, this information was provided to the Congressional Research Service by the Alzheimer's Association on November 21, 2007.

[38] Ashlen Anderson, *Public Policy Responses to Wandering Behavior*.

[39] On November 1, 2007, the Alzheimer's Association, in partnership with MedicAlert, began to offer a bracelet that also includes information about medical conditions (e.g., medication allergies, diabetes, high blood pressure, etc.) of the individual with Alzheimer's disease or dementia. Each identification bracelet is $40 ($49 with accompanying medical information

for the Safe Return program and MedicAlert program) and a $20 annual renewal fee ($25 to include MedicAlert information).

[40] National Center for Missing Adults, *Overview*, November 29, 2007. (Hereafter referenced National Center for Missing Adults, *Overview*.)

[41] National Center for Missing Adults, "National Missing Persons Organizations Merge," press release, http://www.theyaremissed.org/ncma/content.php?webid=NCMA-LBTH-merger.

[42] NCMEC receives federal funding through the Missing and Exploited Children's Program and other sources. For a full discussion of NCMEC activities, see CRS Report RL34050, *Missing and Exploited Children: Background, Policies, and Issues*, by Adrienne L. Fernandes-Alcantara.

[43] This information was provided to the Congressional Research Service by the National Center for Missing and Exploited Children on April 17, 2007.

[44] This section was co-authored with Kirsten J. Colello, Analyst in Gerontology.

[45] For further information, see CRS Report R40552, *Alert Systems for Missing Adults in Eleven States: Background and Issues for Congress*, by Adrienne L. Fernandes-Alcantara and Kirsten J. Colello; and National Association of States United for Aging and Disabilities, *Silver Alert Initiatives in the States: Protecting Seniors with Cognitive Impairments*, November 11, 2010, http://www.nasuad.org/documentation/nasuad_materials/ Silver%20 Alert%20Updated%20Report_11-9-10.pdf.

[46] AMBER Alert systems are voluntary partnerships among law enforcement agencies, broadcasters, and transportation agencies to activate messages in a targeted area when a child is abducted and believed to be in grave danger. For additional information, see CRS Report RL34050, *Missing and Exploited Children: Background, Policies, and Issues*, by Adrienne L. Fernandes-Alcantara.

[47] This information is primarily based on the Congressional Research Service's review of authorizing legislation.

[48] Ashlen Anderson, *Public Policy Responses to Wandering Behavior*.

[49] For example, one such approach might be providing support to the caregivers of individuals with dementia, to better ensure that adults with the disease do not go missing. For information about current federal funding to assist caregivers, see CRS Report RL34123, *Family Caregiving to the Older Population: Background, Federal Programs, and Issues for Congress*, by Kirsten J. Colello.

[50] This information was provided to the Congressional Research Service by Project Lifesaver on March 18, 2008.

[51] For further information, see http://www.projectlifesaver.org/site/.

[52] This information was provided to the Congressional Research Service by the National Center for Missing and Exploited Children on October 25, 2007.

INDEX

A

B

C

D

E

F

G

H

I

J

K

L

M

N

O

PULMONARY AND RESPIRATORY DISEASES AND DISORDERS

ASTHMA

CAUSES, COMPLICATIONS AND TREATMENT

Pulmonary and Respiratory Diseases and Disorders

Additional books in this series can be found on Nova's website under the Series tab.

Additional E-books in this series can be found on Nova's website under the E-book tab.

PULMONARY AND RESPIRATORY DISEASES AND DISORDERS

ASTHMA

CAUSES, COMPLICATIONS AND TREATMENT

ADELINA H. BISLIMI
AND
LULEZIME C. TOLKA
EDITORS

Nova Science Publishers, Inc.
New York

For permission to use material from this book please contact us:
Telephone 631-231-7269; Fax 631-231-8175
Web Site: http://www.novapublishers.com

Library of Congress Cataloging-in-Publication Data

Library of Congress Control Number: 2012941955

ISBN: 978-1-62257-447-6

Published by Nova Science Publishers, Inc. ✝ New York

Contents

Preface

Asthma is a complex disorder characterized by variable and recurring symptoms, airflow obstruction, bronchial hyper-responsiveness, and underlying inflammation. Although asthma is commonly thought of as a disease of children and young adults, a significant percentage of the older adult population is affected and carry a higher rate of morbidity and mortality from the disease. This book examines the causes, complications and treatment of asthma with topics including mathematical modeling in aspirin-induced asthma; the role of neuroimmune and psychological systems in the pathophysiology of bronchial asthma; special considerations of asthma in older adults; changes in the respiratory epithelium in bronchial asthma; and epidemiology of asthma during pregnancy.

Chapter I - It is generally known that leukotrienes and prostaglandins, the products of arachidonic acid (AA) metabolism, play a central role in the pathophysiology of asthma. Cysteinyl leukotrienes (cysLTs) are potent pro-inflammatory mediators that are produced by inflammatory cells and cause bronchoconstriction. Eicosanoid production is strongly dependent on the expressions of the key enzymes in AA metabolic pathways and it is particularly important in the pathophysiological condition called aspirin-induced asthma, in which asthmatic attacks can be induced by ingestion of non-steroidal anti-inflammatory drugs (NSAIDs). It has been recently shown that there exist a strong relationship between the occurrence of aspirin-induced asthma and the expressions of enzymes prostaglandin H synthases 1 and 2 (PGHS1 and PGHS2) as well as leukotriene C_4 synthase (LTC_4S). Several researchers try to distinguish between aspirin -tolerant and -intolerant asthmatics by comparing the expressions of these enzymes. On the other hand, there is a group of researchers who try to explain the occurrence of aspirin-induced asthma *via* the measurements of cysLTs and anti-inflammatory prostaglandins (aiPGs) and by comparisons of their relative productions after NSAID ingestion. According to their hypothesis, the possibility of asthmatic attack largely increases when the production of cysLTs is higher than that of aiPGs.

The aim of our study is to link both experimental approaches by mathematical modeling and computer simulations of eicosanoids production in inflammatory cells in the presence or absence of different NSAIDs. Our approach is systems biology approach in which the knowledge of enzyme gene expressions, molecular interactions, pharmacokinetics of drugs and their action on the molecular level as well as implications on the organ level are integrated. The model enables simulations of different NSAIDs, exogenous PGE_2 analogues, as well as other drugs used in asthma, such as 5-lipoxygenase (5-LOX) inhibitors (5-LOXIBs) and selective PGHS2 inhibitors (coxib-s). The impacts of different enzyme expressions on the production of cysLTs and aiPGs in healthy humans as well as in aspirin -tolerant and -intolerant asthmatics are studied. The results of our model identify alterations in expressions of enzymes PGHS1 and LTC_4S as the key elements in explaining bronchoconstriction, whereas alterations in expression of the enzyme PGHS2 could be linked to other symptoms of aspirin-induced asthma. The model is further used for identification of susceptible patient populations for different NSAIDs and for identification of threshold doses that induce bronchoconstriction. The model predicts the time between NSAID ingestion and bronchoconstriction as well as the duration of symptoms for different NSAID doses. A computer simulation of a strategy for safe NSAIDs administration to aspirin-intolerant asthmatic patients is also proposed and evaluated. Finally, a link between our two cell-type mathematical models, i.e. of eicosanoids production in inflammatory cells and Ca^{2+}-dependent force development in airway smooth muscle cells, will be shortly presented and the missing parts in the present knowledge between these two signaling pathways will be discussed.

Chapter II - Bronchial asthma (BA) is a pathologic disorder, characterized by reversible obstruction, bronchial inflammation and hyperreactivity, bronchial mucus secretion, systemic and local eosinophilia, as well as increased IgE level in serum. Apart from immune mechanisms, several researches point out that asthmatics could be distinguished by a psychological profile described as halfway between patients with mood disorders or anxiety and general population. In addition, the BA or allergic airway inflammation in experimental animals are associated with induction of pro-inflammatory neurotrophins or neuropeptides such as nerve growth factor (NGF), tachykinin peptides substance P (SP) and neurokinin A in bronchoalveolar lavage or nodose sensory neurons innervating lower airways. Using retrograde neuronal tracing technique in combination with double-labeling immunohistochemistry, the allergic sensitization of these animals has been associated with an induction of tachykinin predominantly in airway-specific large-sized (myelinated) jugular–nodose ganglia neurons. Similar changes with respect to neurotrophin / tachykinin labeling are reported in the limbic system after stress-related experiments, while the increased seric level of mentioned neuropeptides is associated with anxious or depressive disorders. These findings suggest that allergen sensitization / challenge (as well as stressful events) may lead to the *de novo* induction of tachykinins in neurons probably via epigenetic mechanisms, putting neuropsychological system of affected subject in a defensive alarming state. It could be concluded that besides the use of bronchodilators and anti-inflammatory medications, the pharmacologic depletion of neuroimmune mechanisms and the consideration of the BA as a psychosomatic and depressive-associated disorder ("bronchial hysteria") may improve the therapeutic approaches in the future.

Chapter III - Asthma is a complex disorder characterized by variable and recurring symptoms of airflow obstruction, bronchial hyperresponsiveness, and underlying inflammation. Although asthma is commonly thought of as a disease of children and young adults, a significant percentage (4-13%) of the older adult (>65 years old) population in the United States is affected and carry a higher rate of morbidity and mortality from the disease. Despite this relatively large prevalence, asthma is often underdiagnosed and undertreated in older adults. The diagnosis of asthma in older adults is challenging due to comorbid conditions and the broad differential diagnosis of other diseases that can produce symptoms similar to asthma. Moreover, older adults have diminished lung and immune function, which can further complicate the disease. A comprehensive assessment that focuses on these issues is necessary to improve the diagnosis and guide therapeutic interventions in older asthmatics. Finally, there are complexities in the management of asthma that are unique to older adults, including the adverse effects of medications, the potential for drug interactions and the paucity of controlled studies examining the efficacy of current asthma treatments in older adults.

Chapter IV - Airway epithelium lines the upper part of the respiratory tract and functions to maintain airway integrity by providing both a physical barrier to inhaled noxious agents and a mechanism for their clearance via the mucociliary escalator. Ciliated columnar cells and goblet cells are the most important cell types in the normal respiratory epithelium. The other types of cells are represented by basal cells, brush cells and Kulchitsky cells (small granule cells). The normal architecture and function of airway epithelium is disturbed in chronic airway inflammatory diseases such as bronchial asthma. Airway remodeling is the general description for the thickening and restructuring of the airways seen in asthma patients. The characteristics of airway remodeling include inflammatory cell infiltration in lamina propria, subepithelial fibrosis, muscular and glandular hypertrophy, thickening of basement membrane and increased vascularity. Damage to the airway epithelium is one prominent feature of bronchial asthma. Epithelium damage includes gap openings, partial or total denudation, goblet cell metaplasia. The increased production of mucus can lead to the formation of plugs that contribute to airway obstruction. Mucin glycoproteins (MUC) are the major macromolecular component of mucus in normal airway epithelium. An increased expression of MUC2, MUC4 and MUC5B has been reported in asthmatic bronchial biopsies. At the epithelium level, in patients with bronchial asthma, appears an increased expression of Ki-67, p21 (WAF1) and decreased expression of FasL, Bcl-2 or Bax, too. Apoptosis of the airway epithelium is increasingly recognized as a potential mechanism by which damage may occur. More work is now needed to comprehend all aspects of this disease, including minimizing the ongoing damage to airway epithelium and consequent airway remodeling.

Chapter V - Chronic bronchial asthma is the most commonly encountered respiratory disorder complicating pregnancy and is a potentially serious medical condition that represents a significant public health issue. The prevalence of asthma in pregnant women ranges between 0.4% and 12% (with an average of 4–8%) and appears to have increased over recent decades. Kwon et al. demonstrated a two-fold increase in the prevalence of asthma from 2.9% to 5.8% between 1976–1980 and 1988–1994. This diversity of statistics is presumably the result of differences in the definitions of asthma.

In: Asthma: Causes, Complications and Treatment ISBN: 978-1-62257-447-6
Editors: A. H. Bislimi and L. C. Tolka

Chapter I

Mathematical Modeling in Aspirin-Induced Asthma: Theory and Clinical Applications

Aleš Fajmut[1], Andrej Dobovišek[1] and Milan Brumen[1,2]
[1] University of Maribor, Faculty of Natural Sciences and Mathematics, Faculty of Medicine, Faculty of Health Sciences, Maribor, Slovenia
[2] Institute Jožef Stefan, Ljubljana, Slovenia

Abstract

It is generally known that leukotrienes and prostaglandins, the products of arachidonic acid (AA) metabolism, play a central role in the pathophysiology of asthma. Cysteinyl leukotrienes (cysLTs) are potent pro-inflammatory mediators that are produced by inflammatory cells and cause bronchoconstriction. Eicosanoid production is strongly dependent on the expressions of the key enzymes in AA metabolic pathways and it is particularly important in the pathophysiological condition called aspirin-induced asthma, in which asthmatic attacks can be induced by ingestion of non-steroidal anti-inflammatory drugs (NSAIDs). It has been recently shown that there exist a strong relationship between the occurrence of aspirin-induced asthma and the expressions of enzymes prostaglandin H synthases 1 and 2 (PGHS1 and PGHS2) as well as leukotriene C_4 synthase (LTC_4S). Several researchers try to distinguish between aspirin -tolerant and -intolerant asthmatics by comparing the expressions of these enzymes. On the other hand, there is a group of researchers who try to explain the occurrence of aspirin-induced asthma *via* the measurements of cysLTs and anti-inflammatory prostaglandins (aiPGs) and by comparisons of their relative productions after NSAID ingestion. According to their hypothesis, the possibility of asthmatic attack largely increases when the production of cysLTs is higher than that of aiPGs.

The aim of our study is to link both experimental approaches by mathematical modeling and computer simulations of eicosanoids production in inflammatory cells in the presence or absence of different NSAIDs. Our approach is systems biology approach in which the knowledge of enzyme gene expressions, molecular interactions, pharmacokinetics of drugs and their action on the molecular level as well as implications on the organ level are integrated. The model enables simulations of different NSAIDs, exogenous PGE_2 analogues, as well as other drugs used in asthma, such as 5-lipoxygenase (5-LOX) inhibitors (5-LOXIBs) and selective PGHS2 inhibitors (coxib-s). The impacts of different enzyme expressions on the production of cysLTs and aiPGs in healthy humans as well as in aspirin -tolerant and -intolerant asthmatics are studied. The results of our model identify alterations in expressions of enzymes PGHS1 and LTC_4S as the key elements in explaining bronchoconstriction, whereas alterations in expression of the enzyme PGHS2 could be linked to other symptoms of aspirin-induced asthma. The model is further used for identification of susceptible patient populations for different NSAIDs and for identification of threshold doses that induce bronchoconstriction. The model predicts the time between NSAID ingestion and bronchoconstriction as well as the duration of symptoms for different NSAID doses. A computer simulation of a strategy for safe NSAIDs administration to aspirin-intolerant asthmatic patients is also proposed and evaluated. Finally, a link between our two cell-type mathematical models, i.e. of eicosanoids production in inflammatory cells and Ca^{2+}-dependent force development in airway smooth muscle cells, will be shortly presented and the missing parts in the present knowledge between these two signaling pathways will be discussed.

Introduction

Asthma is an inflammatory condition of the airways characterized by airway smooth muscle hyperreactivity and hypersensitivity, excessive secretion of mucus, and multicellular inflammation involving activated mast cells, eosinophils, neutrophils, macrophages, basophils, and lymphocytes [1]. In a subset of asthmatic patients, exposure to aspirin and other non-steroidal anti-inflammatory drugs (NSAIDs) temporarily accentuate the inflammatory process, leading to asthma exacerbations [1]. This distinct clinical syndrome that affects around 10-20 % of asthmatic patients is usually called aspirin-induced asthma. Many other terms have been used to describe this respiratory disease: aspirin-sensitive asthma, aspirin hypersensitivity, aspirin idiosyncrasy, aspirin intolerance and aspirin-exacerbated respiratory disease (AERD) [2]. All terms refer to the same disease and the same patients who are afflicted with instantaneous inflammation of both - upper and lower - respiratory tracts accompanied by bronchoconstriction, rhino-sinusitis, swollen eyes, urticaria as well as flushing head and neck after ingestion of typical NSAID doses. The symptoms usually occur 30-60 min after NSAID ingestion [2] and can last up to 9 hours [3].

The process of distinguishing between aspirin-intolerant (AIA) and aspirin-tolerant (ATA) asthmatic patients is performed with provocation tests, in which patients are challenged with different doses of NSAIDs by either ingestion or inhalation. In order to follow the level of bronchoconstriction, FEV_1 is measured. Finally, threshold doses, above which patients react with bronchoconstriction, are determined for each particular NSAID [4]. However, all AIA patients do not undergo bronchoconstrictive reaction after NSAID dosing and thus, the observations of skin reactions, quick- and long- term nasal responses to NSAIDs are necessary. When AIA patients undergo challenges with NSAIDs, very substantial increases in urinary LTE_4 levels and decreases in PGE_2 are recorded during bronchospastic reactions [5] or nasal responses [6]. Increases in LTC_4 and histamine levels in both nasal [7] and bronchial [8] fluids after oral aspirin challenges have also been detected in AIA.

Long term follow-up of AIA patients are nasal polyps, which may occur even ten years after first short-term reactions to NSAIDs [9]. In 1922, the first article appeared, describing the association of aspirin sensitivity, asthma, and nasal polyposis. In the late 1960s, this clinical entity was named "aspirin triad" [10]. In the last years, chronic hyperplastic eosinophilic sinusitis (CHES) became known as the fourth remarkable symptom of aspirin induced asthma [11].

Aspirin-induced asthma is a major medical problem but, despite decades of research, the exact mechanisms that underlie this condition remain unclear. An unsolved question in the research of aspirin-induced asthma still remains, why ingestion of NSAIDs does not induce bronchoconstrictive reactions and other symptoms in all humans, or at least in all asthmatic patients [11].

Pathogenesis of Aspirin-Induced Asthma

The main role in the occurrence of aspirin-induced asthma is attributed to the increase of the production of cysteinyl leukotrienes (cysLTs) - metabolites of arachidonic acid (AA) that are mainly produced in epithelial cells and in leukocytes, involved in inflammation [2, 11]. Among all leukotrienes (LT), LTC_4 is the most potent mediator of asthma and inflammation. It induces bronchoconstriction and inflammatory cell recruitment in asthmatic patients as well as in healthy humans [12]. It is a product of lipoxygenase pathway of AA degradation, in which AA is first transformed into leukotriene A_4 (LTA_4) by the enzyme 5-lipoxygenase (5-LOX) *via* short-lived intermediate product 5-hydroperoxyeicosatetraenoic acid (5-HETE) (see Figure 1). Then LTA_4 is further transformed into leukotriene B_4 (LTB_4) by the enzyme LTA_4 hydrolase (LTA_4H) or it is conjugated with glutathione (GSH) into LTC_4 by the enzyme leukotriene C_4 synthase (LTC_4S). In the latter enzymatic reaction, LTA_4 is involved as a substrate and LTC_4 as a product, whereby LTA_4 auto-regulates the velocity of its own degradation [13]. Both leukotrienes LTB_4 and LTC_4 are then exported to extracellular space, whereby LTC_4 is first transformed to LTD_4 and later to LTE_4. The latter three represent a group of cysteinyl leukotrienes (cysLT). LTE_4 is usually found and measured in urine [6, 14]. All cysLTs can bind to two types of G-protein coupled transmembrane receptors, $cysLT_1R$ and $cysLT_2R$, of bronchial smooth muscles, and induce contraction. With respect to other inhaled contractile agonists, LTC_4 and LTD_4 are approximately 3,000-times and LTE_4 approximately 30-times more potent than histamine as bronchoconstrictor agonists in healthy humans [15]. Maximal bronchoconstrictive response to LTD_4 is even greater than that to methacholine [15].

In the second pathway of AA degradation, cyclooxygenase pathway (see Figure 1), AA is transformed into anti- (aiPGs) and pro-(piPGs) inflammatory prostaglandins by the enzymes prostaglandin H synthase 1 (PGHS1) and prostaglandin H synthase 2 (PGHS2), often referred to as cyclooxygenase 1 (COX-1) and cyclooxygenase 2 (COX-2) [18]. PGE_2 is the most important representative of aiPGs. In many cells, including endothelial and epithelial cells of the respiratory tract, it has profound regulatory effects: (1) it reduces LT biosynthesis through inhibition of 5-LOX [14, 19, 20]; (2) it prevents discharge of granular mediators from lung mast cells [21]; and (3) it prevents bronchoconstriction [14, 22]. Underproduction of PGE_2 strongly diminishes the inhibitory effects of PGE_2 on 5-LOX, thus, enhances cysLT production, and reduces the inhibitory effect of PGE_2 on mast cells, releasing histamine and tryptase [21, 23, 24]. In this way, decreased levels of PGE_2 might induce bronchoconstriction.

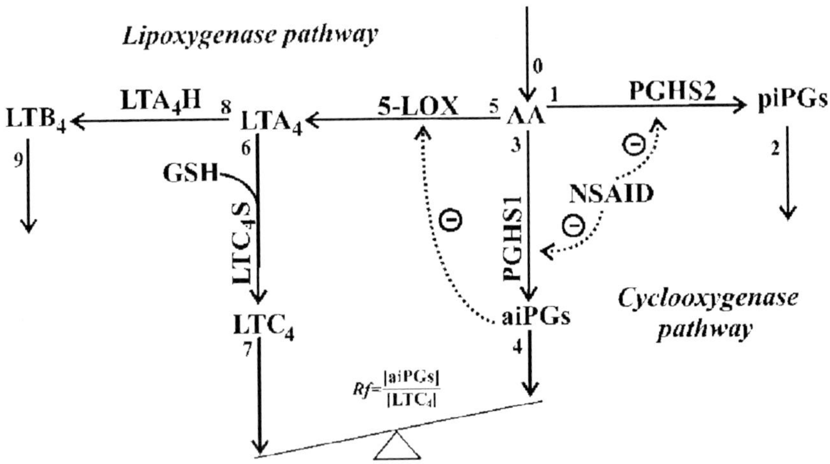

Figure 1. General scheme of eicosanoid production pathways of arachidonic acid (AA) metabolism considered for mathematical modeling. Similar kinetic scheme was considered in our previous publications [16, 17]. Action of NSAID and 5-LOX inhibitors (5-LOXIB) is indicated. The balance between aiPGs and LTC_4 production is schematically presented. Numeration of the fluxes is in accordance with the reaction velocities of the mathematical model.

The balance between synthesis of prostaglandins and leukotrienes (see Figure 1) mainly depends on the production of PGE_2 by the inhibition, which PGE_2 exerts on 5-LOX [14, 19, 20]. The target of inhibitory action of PGE_2 is 5-LOX activating protein (FLAP); however, the entire mechanism of this inhibition is not completely revealed [2, 20, 25]. The majority of NSAIDs inhibit both enzymes of cyclooxygenase pathway, PGHS1 and PGHS2 [26, 27], reduce the total prostaglandin production and, thus, also lower the synthesis of PGE_2 [28]. The decrease in PGE_2 synthesis reduces the inhibitory effect on 5-LOX, which leads to enhanced synthesis of cysLTs [2, 20, 28]. This seems to be the critical event that tilts AA metabolism in favor of the lipoxygenase pathway and leads to overproduction of LTC_4. However, this mechanism does not explain the different effects of NSAIDs on AIA patients from the ones that are present in ATA patients or healthy humans (HH).

Aspirin, indomethacin and ibuprofen, for example, inhibit both enzymes but are much more potent inhibitors of PGHS1 than PGHS2 [11]. From clinical practice it is known that these NSAIDs precipitate asthmatic attacks in AIA patients already at low doses [11]. Aspirin (80%) and ibuprofen (41%) were the most commonly reported NSAIDs to elicit prior respiratory reactions [29], and ibuprofen is a drug which was most often confirmed as being the cause of NSAID intolerance [30]. Nimesulide and meloxicam, drugs known to inhibit PGHS2 substantially more than PGHS1 (they are 5-50 -times more selective for PGHS2 than PGHS1), are well tolerated by AIA when given average therapeutic doses, but cause rhinorrhea and mild asthma attacks when ingested in higher doses (e.g. 15 mg of meloxicam) [31, 32]. More recently, several highly selective inhibitors of PGHS2, such as celecoxib, rofecoxib, etoricoxib, parecoxib, lumiracoxib, valedcoxib, were introduced into clinical practice [11]. The idea behind these selective inhibitors is that they inhibit PGHS1 much less than PGHS2 and, in this way, do not reduce inhibitory action of PGE_2 on 5-LOX and, consequently, do not increase LTC_4 levels. As such they should theoretically be safe for AIA patients. In the large majority of studies with these selective drugs, at doses even higher than therapeutic, none of AIA patients reacted to them [33-38]. Although few studies report respiratory reactions to selective PGHS2 inhibitors [39], these drugs still carry the warning label "aspirin triad" as a contraindication and only celecoxib is available in the United States market [2]. Later in this chapter, we will present theoretically predicted limiting doses of celecoxib that represent the limit, above which this drug might potentially induce bronchoconstriction in different AIA patient populations.

A special role for PGE_2 has been attributed to the pathogenesis of AIA [40]. Peripheral blood macrophage cells of some patients with AIA synthesize less PGE_2 at baseline than normal [41]. This disadvantage of lacking sufficient concentrations of cellular or transcellular PGE_2 leads to overproduction of LTs. There is clear evidence that many, but not all, AIA patients synthesize excessive amounts of cysLTs, before and after exposure to NSAIDs [5, 42]. It is believed that aspirin-induced asthma is largely attributed to LTC_4 overproduction. Limitation of cysLT production is possible by inhibitors of 5-LOX, such as zileuton and ABT-761 [43, 44]. Efficacy of zileuton, most known inhibitor of 5-LOX, has been demonstrated in clinical study [42] and zileuton is in addition to $cysLT_1R$ antagonists ($cysLT_1RA$) (e.g. montelukast, zafirlukast, pranlukast) most frequently used in preventing bronchospastic reactions during oral aspirin challenges [2]. As an example, we will present theoretically predicted strategy for potentially safe administration of ABT-761 and ibuprofen together to different AIA patient populations and the differences that might occur between these populations. Such strategies are common when

NSAIDs should be administered to AIA patients because of their other health problems, such as chronic headaches or rheumatic arthritis, for example [45].

In *in-vitro* tests it was evidenced that the effect of exogenous PGE_2 is a reduction of cysLT production in the inflammatory cells from mucosa of human bronchial biopsies [46]. It was also shown that exogenous PGE_2 results in attenuation of the physiologic early and late asthmatic responses. Its main role, either by exogenous administration or by increase in endogenous production, is the protective anti-inflammatory management of allergic asthma in the early phase of asthmatic response [47]. The protective effects of exogenous PGE_2 were studied and confirmed in humans with asthma, induced by NSAIDs [14], allergens [47, 48] or exercise [49]. In all these cases, PGE_2 was administered by inhalation in form of aerosol. Similarly, misoprostol, the oral-stable analogue of PGE_1, also attenuated bronchoconstriction precipitated by aspirin, although its potency was weaker than that of inhaled PGE_2 [36]. The use of nocloprost, an oral-stable form of PGE_2, which is mainly used as a protective prostaglandin in treatment of NSAID-induced gastric ulcers [50], was also proposed for the treatment of AIA [41]. In our recent study [17], we proposed a strategy on the basis of our mathematical model for safe administration of oral stable PGE_2 analogue – nocloprost in combination with either aspirin or ibuprofen to different AIA patient populations. In this chapter, we will summarize our findings and compare this strategy with the one, carried out with ABT-761.

PGE_2 is mainly produced by the enzyme PGHS1 in the cyclooxygenase pathway of AA degradation [2]. Thus, its production rate strongly depends on the enzyme availability. PGHS1 is a constitutively expressed enzyme that is present in most mammalian cells, including respiratory epithelial cells, as well as inflammatory cells. PGHS2 is expressed mainly in respiratory epithelium and in inflammatory cells and it is an inducible enzyme that is highly upregulated by pro-inflammatory mediators [2]. In bronchi of patients with stable asthma and chronic bronchitis, these two enzymes are not quantitatively up- or down- regulated, but there is evidence that expression of PGHS2 is diminished and its activity is reduced in AIA patients [51, 52]. Reference [51] reports 6-fold lower expression of PGHS2 in nasal polyps and nasal mucosa of AIA patients compared to ATA. Reference [53] reports 3-fold lower expression of PGHS1 in bronchial fibroblasts in AIA patients, compared to those in ATA. Other authors did not observe any significant differences in overall expressions of PGHS1 and PGHS2 in bronchial biopsy specimens, obtained from ATA and AIA patients [54, 55]. Many, but not all, AIA patients demonstrate overexpression of LTC_4S in eosinophils and mast cells in their bronchial biopsy specimens, and in circulating eosinophils [54, 56, 57]. References [11, 54] report 5-fold higher expression of LTC_4S in AIA compared to ATA patients as well as 20-fold higher expression in AIA compared to healthy humans (HH) in bronchial biopsy specimens. These differences between AIA and ATA patients and HH in the expressions of the key enzymes of AA degradation are the basis for the definition of our different model populations. In our recently published work [16], we defined five different model populations. Three of them represent three different aspirin-intolerant asthmatic patient populations ($AIA^{(1)}$, $AIA^{(2)}$, $AIA^{(3)}$), one determines aspirin-tolerant asthmatics (ATA) and another one determines healthy humans (HH).

Common features that are emerging throughout most experimental studies, supposedly grouping AIA patients into subgroups, are that AIA patients produce more LTC_4 and less PGE_2 than ATA and HH. Moreover, they have upregulated expressions of $cysLT_1R$ [58] and LTC_4S [11, 54, 56, 57] and downregulated expressions of E-series prostanoid 2 (EP2) and 3 (EP3) receptors [59], as well as of PGHS1 and PGHS2 [51-53, 55] in their inflammatory cells. However, clear separation between AIA and ATA patient groups has not been accomplished in experimental procedures because of the considerable overlapping between the groups in their inflammatory profiles [5]. To make matters more difficult, different AIA patients present distinct symptoms of AIA and their clinical presentation of the disease can be mild, moderate, or severe [5]. Despite that, a pattern is emerging in which many defects in either overstimulation of inflammation or underproduction of anti-inflammatory mediators as well as overproduction of pro-inflammatory mediators and bronchoconstrictors, especially in the eicosanoid family, is found in AIA patients [2]. One of such patterns occurred in the study [41], of which the long term goal was to check the possibility of a simple and cheap *in-vitro* whole blood test for routine diagnosis of aspirin intolerance. Authors of that study observed that selected AIA patients, who had bronchoconstrictive reactions after aspirin inhalation, produced higher amounts of LTC_4 than PGE_2 after NSAID exposure. They introduced the concept of the relation factor (*Rf*), defined as the ratio between PGE_2 and LTC_4 concentrations in peripheral blood cells [41]. *Rf* is for AIA patients with bronchoconstrictive reactions lower than one, whereas for ATA patients as well as healthy humans (HH) it is always more than one [41]. In our model simulations, we use relation factor as a quantitative criterion in predicting bronchoconstriction, limiting drug doses and the strategies for safe drug administration. We defined it as the ratio between the concentrations of aiPGs and LTC_4 [16].

In spite of accumulating and promising experimental and clinical results, as shortly introduced in this chapter above, molecular and cellular mechanism of inducing and developing processes in aspirin induced asthma, pushing the asthmatics to the risk and likely to bronchospastic reactions, are still not completely revealed and understood. It is obvious that experimental and clinical research is running on different molecular, cellular and organ levels as well as on the multiscale level. Our work presented in this chapter is a theoretical contribution to these investigations. A theoretical analysis and predictions attained from mathematical modeling can combine the different levels of investigation and serve for formulation of the framework of experimental observations. In short, the gene and molecular level yields analysis of gene expression for the key enzymes involved in AA metabolism and the search for their genetic polymorphisms as well as the search for overexpression of cysLTR and underexpression of EP2 and EP3 receptors; the cellular-tissue level covers measurements of the inflammatory profiles in terms of eicosanoid production in particular cells and tissues before and after NSAID exposure; and the tissue, organ or organism level is the level of observations of the symptoms of AIA and bronchospastic reactions.

Mathematical Model and Model Populations

The kinetic scheme of AA metabolism and its interaction with NSAID and 5 LOX inhibitor is given in Fig. 1, which was also considered for mathematical modeling in our previous publications [16, 17]. The basic entity of the corresponding mathematical model is a set of six first-order ordinary differential equations, describing the time evolution of system variables, which are concentrations of metabolites as follows: $[AA]$, $[piPGs]$, $[aiPGs]$, $[LTA_4]$, $[LTB_4]$ and $[LTC_4]$, i= 1…6, respectively :

$$\frac{d[S_i]}{dt} = \sum_{\text{incoming}} v_k - \sum_{\text{outgoing}} v_l \qquad (1)$$

The time evolution of a selected system variable $[S_i]$ is taken into account as the difference between the sum of all incoming and the sum of all outgoing metabolic fluxes, both with respect to numeration in the kinetic scheme in Fig. 1. v_k and v_l are also known as reaction velocities.

Reaction velocity v_0 represents the cell influx of AA and its value is taken to be constant in all simulations, v_0=0.7 μMs^{-1}. Reaction velocity v_1 describes the enzyme PGHS2 with the steady-state Michaelis-Menten expression, which takes into account interactions of the enzyme with substrate AA and inhibitor NSAID [27, 60]:

$$v_1 = \frac{v_{\max 1}[AA]}{K_1\left(1+\frac{[NSAID]}{K_{I1}^{(j)}}\right)+[AA]}, \tag{2}$$

where $v_{\max 1}$ is the maximal velocity of the reaction, K_1 is the Michaelis-Menten constant and K_{I1} is the equilibrium dissociation constant of inhibitory action of NSAID on PGHS2. Superscript (j) denotes the type of the drug, which is one of NSAIDs (either aspirin, $j=ASA$, ibuprofen, $j=IBU$ or celecoxib, $j=CEL$). Reaction velocity v_2, i.e. the piPGs efflux, is described as [61]:

$$v_2 = k_2[piPGs], \tag{3}$$

where k_2 is the reaction rate constant. Reaction velocity v_3 of the enzyme PGHS1 is described as [27, 60]:

$$v_3 = \frac{v_{\max 3}[AA]}{K_3\left(1+\frac{[NSAID]}{K_{I3}^{(j)}}\right)+[AA]}, \tag{4}$$

where $v_{\max 3}$ is the maximal velocity of the reaction and K_3 is the Michaelis-Menten constant.

K_{I3} is the equilibrium dissociation constant of inhibitory action of NSAID on PGHS1. Superscript (j) denotes the type of the drug, which is one of NSAIDs (either aspirin, $j=ASA$, ibuprofen, $j=IBU$ or celecoxib, $j=CEL$). Reaction velocity v_4 is considered as [61]:

$$v_4 = k_4[aiPGs], \tag{5}$$

where k_4 is the rate constant for aiPGs efflux from the cell. Reaction velocity v_5 describes degradation of AA by the enzyme 5-LOX in terms of Michaelis-Menten kinetics, whereby inhibitory actions of aiPGs and 5-LOX inhibitors (5-LOXIB) on 5-LOX are considered [62]:

$$v_5 = \frac{v_{\max 5}[AA]}{K_5(1+\frac{[aiPGs_{TOT}]}{K_{I5}}+\frac{[5-LOXIB]}{K_{I5}^{(j)}})+[AA]}, \tag{6}$$

where $v_{\max 5}$ is the maximal velocity of the reaction, K_5 is the Michaelis-Menten constant and K_{I5}, $K_{I5}^{(j)}$ are the equilibrium constants of inhibitory action of total aiPGs (both, native and administered) as well as of other 5-LOX inhibitors, acting in parallel with aiPGs, on 5-LOX, respectively. Superscript (j) denotes the type of 5-LOXIB, which is ABT-761 (j=ABT) in one of the simulations. Reaction velocity v_6 describes the mechanism of LTC_4 production, in which LTA_4 and glutathione (GSH) are conjugated with LTC_4S:

$$v_6 = \frac{v_{\max 6}[LTA_4]}{A+B[LTA_4]+C[LTA_4]^2}, \tag{7}$$

A, B and C are the parameters and $v_{\max 6}$ is the maximal reaction velocity. Reaction velocity v_7 describes the efflux of LTC_4 from the cell [63]

$$v_7 = k_7[LTC_4], \tag{8}$$

where $k_7$is the reaction rate constant. Reaction velocity v_8 describes conversion of LTA_4 into LTB_4 by the enzyme LTA_4H as [64]:

$$v_8 = \frac{v_{\max 8}[LTA_4]}{K_8+[LTA_4]}, \tag{9}$$

and reaction velocity v_9 describes efflux of LTB_4 from cells by [65]:

$$v_9 = \frac{v_{\max 9}[LTB_4]}{K_9+[LTB_4]}. \tag{10}$$

In both above equations the meaning of parameters is the same as above.

Time courses of drug concentrations in the plasma are described by the standard pharmacokinetic model that takes into account absorption and elimination phases of the drug:

$$[DRUG] = \frac{D^{(j)} k_a^{(j)}}{(V/F)^{(j)} \left(k_a^{(j)} - k_e^{(j)}\right)} \left(e^{-k_e^{(j)} t} - e^{-k_a^{(j)} t}\right), \tag{11}$$

where $D^{(j)}$ is the drug dose, $(V/F)^{(j)}$ is the ratio between apparent volume of drug distribution and fraction of the drug absorbed, $k_a^{(j)}$ and $k_e^{(j)}$ are the first order absorption and elimination rate constants, respectively. [*DRUG*] is [*NSAID*] and/or [*5-LOXIB*]. Superscript (*j*) denotes the type of the drug, which is one of NSAIDs (either aspirin, j=*ASA*, ibuprofen, j=*IBU* or celecoxib, j=*CEL*) and/or 5-LOXIBs (ABT-761, j=*ABT*).

Total aiPGs concentration $[aiPGs_{\mathrm{TOT}}]$ is given by the equation:

$$[aiPGs_{\mathrm{TOT}}] = [aiPGs] + \frac{D^{(PGE)} k_a^{(PGE)}}{(V/F)^{(PGE)} (k_a^{(PGE)} - k_e^{(PGE)})} (e^{-k_e^{(PGE)} t} - e^{-k_a^{(PGE)} t}). \tag{12}$$

The first term in the above equation considers aiPGs produced in the cell and the second term describes the level of exogenous PGE_2 analogue, administered orally to the patient, by the absorption and elimination phases. We consider the inhibitory effect of endogenous and exogenous PGE_2 on 5-LOX to be the same since there is strong evidence that PGE_2 exerts the inhibition in an autocrine manner [20, 25, 47].

Relation factor (*Rf*) is according to [41] defined as:

$$Rf = \frac{[aiPGs_{\mathrm{TOT}}]}{[LTC_4]}, \tag{13}$$

and is a measure of critical conditions for the risk of bronchoconstriction in AIA patients. In accordance with the experimental findings [41], bronchoconstriction occurs when $Rf<1$. Descriptions of the model parameters and their values, used in our previous [16, 17] and present model simulations are given in Tables 1 and 2. Model parameters v_{max1}, v_{max3} and v_{max6} are defined and described later in this chapter.

Table 1. Kinetic parameters used in model simulations

Parameter	Value and unit	Description	References
v_0	0.7 μMs^{-1}	AA influx	[16, 17]
K_1	2.5 μM	Michaelis-Menten constant	[66]
$K_{I1}^{(ASA)}$	85 μM	equilibrium dissociation constant of inhibitory action of aspirin on PGHS2	[67]
$K_{I1}^{(IBU)}$	60 μM	equilibrium dissociation constant of inhibitory action of ibuprofen on PGHS2	[67]
$K_{I1}^{(CEL)}$	0.07 μM	equilibrium dissociation constant of inhibitory action of celecoxib on PGHS2	[68]
k_2	0.0028 s^{-1}	rate constant of piPGs efflux	[61]
K_3	3.0 μM	Michaelis-Menten constant	[66]
$K_{I3}^{(ASA)}$	4.0 μM	equilibrium dissociation constant of inhibitory action of aspirin on PGHS1	[67]
$K_{I3}^{(IBU)}$	1.3 μM	equilibrium dissociation constant of inhibitory action of ibuprofen on PGHS1	[67]
$K_{I3}^{(CEL)}$	0.2 μM	equilibrium dissociation constant of inhibitory action of celecoxib on PGHS1	[68]
k_4	0.0028 s^{-1}	rate constant of aiPGs efflux	[61]
v_{max5}	86 μMs^{-1}	maximal velocity of reaction	[69]
K_5	25.4 μM	equilibrium dissociation constant	[62]
K_{I5}	0.03 μM	equilibrium dissociation constant of inhibitory action of aiPGs on 5-LOX	[20]
$K_{I5}^{(ABT)}$	0.018 μM	equilibrium dissociation constant of inhibitory action of ABT-761 on 5-LOX	[70]
A	56 μM	constant	[71]
B	1.4	constant	[71]
C	0.17 μM^{-1}	constant	[71]
k_7	0.0015 s^{-1}	rate constant of LTC_4 efflux	[63]
v_{max8}	3.7 μMs^{-1}	maximal velocity of the reaction	[64]
K_8	27 μM	Michaelis-Menten constant	[64]
v_{max9}	5.74 μMs^{-1}	maximal velocity of the reaction	[65]
K_9	239 μM	half-saturation constant	[65]

For theoretical analysis we use three basic populations, healthy humans (HH), aspirin-tolerant (ATA) and aspirin-intolerant (AIA) asthmatic patients, whereby we distinguish and postulate three different AIA model populations: $AIA^{(1)}$, $AIA^{(2)}$ and $AIA^{(3)}$. They are characterized according to experimental findings about the differences in expressions of the key enzymes PGHS2, PGHS1 and LTC_4S [11, 51, 53, 54]. Thus in modeling, the parameters v_{max1},

v_{max3} and v_{max6}, reflecting different expressions of the enzymes PGHS2, PGHS1 and LTC_4S, respectively, are taken as free model parameters and their values were adjusted according to the known experimental data. Hence, AIA model populations differ from each other in the parameter values v_{max1}, v_{max3} and v_{max6}. Direct proportionalities between the expressions of the enzymes and their maximal activities are considered.

Table 2. Values of pharmacokinetic parameters for oral application of aspirin, ibuprofen, PGE_2 analogue – nocloprost and ABT-761. Doses of the drugs ($D^{(j)}$) stand in the text

Parameter	Value and unit	Description	References
ASPIRIN			
$k_e^{(ASA)}$	$5.5 \cdot 10^{-4}$ s^{-1}	elimination rate constant	[72]
$k_a^{(ASA)}$	$23 \cdot 10^{-4}$ s^{-1}	absorption rate constant	[72]
$V/F^{(ASA)}$	74 L	apparent volume of distribution/fraction of aspirin absorbed	[72]
IBUPROFEN			
$k_e^{(IBU)}$	$1.0 \cdot 10^{-4}$ s^{-1}	elimination rate constant	[73]
$k_a^{(IBU)}$	$2.8 \cdot 10^{-4}$ s^{-1}	absorption rate constant	[73]
$V/F^{(IBU)}$	8.4 L	apparent volume of distribution/fraction of ibuprofen absorbed	[73]
CELECOXIB			
$k_e^{(CEL)}$	$4{,}4 \cdot 10^{-5}$ s^{-1}	elimination rate constant	[74]
$k_a^{(CEL)}$	$2.0 \cdot 10^{-4}$ s^{-1}	absorption rate constant	[74]
$V/F^{(CEL)}$	242 L	apparent volume of distribution/fraction of celecoxib absorbed	[74]
PGE_2 ANALOGUE - NOCLOPROST			
$k_e^{(PGE)}$	$3.3 \cdot 10^{-4}$ s^{-1}	elimination rate constant	[50]
$k_a^{(PGE)}$	$8.1 \cdot 10^{-4}$ s^{-1}	absorption rate constant	[50]
$V/F^{(PGE)}$	13 L	apparent volume of distribution/fraction of nocloprost absorbed	[50]
ABT-761			
$k_e^{(ABT)}$	$1.4 \cdot 10^{-5}$ s^{-1}	elimination rate constant	[75]
$k_a^{(ABT)}$	$3.2 \cdot 10^{-4}$ s^{-1}	absorption rate constant	[75]
$V/F^{(ABT)}$	60L	apparent volume of distribution/fraction of ABT-761 absorbed	[75]

Model population ATA represents the reference model population, which was already determined in our previous study [16]. The reference values of model parameters v_{max1}=0.65 μMs^{-1} and v_{max6}=0.23 μMs^{-1} were obtained from experimental studies [27, 71].The value v_{max3}=0,096 μMs^{-1} was determined specifically for ATA by obtaining the best agreement between the model [16] and the experiment [41]. Since the parameter value v_{max3} was determined specifically for ATA patients and all other parameters were determined non-specifically (the experimental studies do not report any pathologies), the whole set of parameter values, v_{max1}=0.65 μMs^{-1}, v_{max3}=0.096 μM and v_{max6}=0.23 μMs^{-1}, defines the model population ATA [16].

Different model AIA patient populations are defined with respect to ATA as follows [16]:

i. AIA$^{(1)}$: with 3-fold decreased expression of the enzyme PGHS1: v_{max1}=0.65 μM, v_{max3}=0.032 μM and v_{max6}=0.23 μM. The reduced PGHS1 activity [41] and 3-fold lower expression of PGHS1 [53], both in AIA patients with respect to ATA patients were observed.
ii. AIA$^{(2)}$: with 5-fold increased expression of the enzyme LTC_4S: v_{max1}=0.65 μM, v_{max3}=0.096 μM and v_{max6}=1.15 μM. 5-fold higher expression of LTC_4S in AIA compared to ATA patients was reported [11, 54].
iii. AIA$^{(3)}$: with 6-fold decreased expression of the enzyme PGHS2: v_{max1}=0.11 μM, v_{max3}=0.096 μM and v_{max6} =0.23 μM. Reference [51] reports 6-fold lower expression of PGHS2 in AIA compared to ATA patients.
iv. HH: with 4-fold decreased expression of the enzyme LTC_4S: v_{max1}=0.65 μM, v_{max3}=0.096 μM and v_{max6} =0.057 μM. References [11, 54] report 20-fold lower expression in HH compared to AIA$^{(2)}$.

Software used for all calculations was Berkeley Madonna 8.0.1 (R. Macey and G. Oster, University of California at Berkeley). The system of differential equations, evolved from equation (1) by considering all definitions of the fluxes and plasma drug distributions, was numerically integrated from the initial stationary state, which was determined for each model variable in the absence of NSAID for each particular model population. In simulations, we used numerical integration method with variable integration step.

Results and Discussion

Clinical signs such as rhinitis, conjunctivitis and bronchoconstriction in AIA usually occur within 30 to 60 min after ingestion of NSAID irrespective of its type [2]. On the other hand, smooth muscle strips contract approximately 15 min after stimulation with LTC_4 [76]. If we add these 15 min to the value of time, at which relation factor *Rf* drops below one after NSAID dosing (typically 20 – 30 min, depending on the type of NSAID, its dose and AIA model population [16]), we get similar time interval (35 – 45 min) as the one observed in clinical tests (30 – 60 min) [2]. Relation factor (*Rf*) was first introduced by Schäfer et al. in 1999 [41]. The authors showed, by simultaneous measurements of FEV_1 and the concentrations of PGE_2 and LTC_4 in peripheral blood cells of AIA patients, that those AIA patients, for which the value of *Rf* is lower than one, might undergo bronchoconstriction with high probability after aspirin dosing [41]. *Rf* is in our model defined as the ratio between concentrations of aiPGs and LTC_4 and is presented in Figure 2 (dash-dot line) along with the time dependencies of aiPGs and LTC_4 concentrations. Simulation is performed for the model population $AIA^{(1)}$, which represents AIA patient population with 3-fold lower expression of PGHS1, and 200 mg dose of ibuprofen applied at time t=0 h.

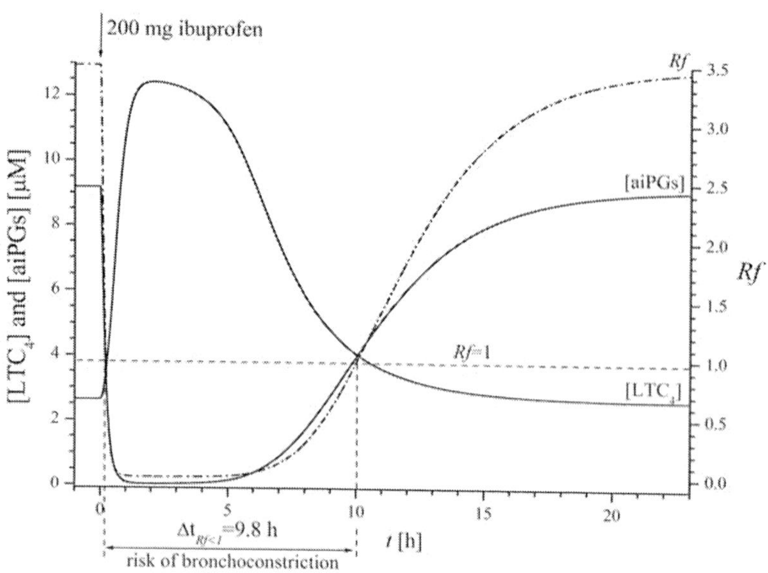

Figure 2. Time course of *[LTC_4]*, *[aiPGs]* and *Rf* after 200 mg ibuprofen dosing.

In Figure 2, the time interval of *Rf*, being less than one, is annotated. Since the value of *Rf* less than one is according to [41] characterized as the state of high risk for bronchoconstriction, the whole time interval is a theoretical estimation for the duration of bronchoconstriction. For the model population $AIA^{(1)}$ and for 200 mg of ibuprofen, the theoretical estimation is 9.8 h. This is in accordance with the value observed in clinical tests (9 h) [3]. Our mathematical model enables the theoretical prediction of NSAID dose for which symptoms of aspirin-induced asthma might appear. We introduced so-called limiting dose, D_{limit}, which could be calculated for any NSAID by knowing its pharmacokinetic parameters and its inhibitory properties on the enzymes PGHS1 and PGHS2. Limiting dose for particular NSAID is determined with the condition $Rf = 1$. D_{limit} is the theoretical estimation for the threshold dose ($D_{treshold}$) that is determined with provocation tests in clinical practice. Threshold dose is the dose of NSAID, used in this test, above which significant bronchoconstriction and other symptoms of aspirin-induced asthma occur in AIA patients. Threshold doses are usually determined by measurements of FEV_1 or by observations of different clinical signs of aspirin-induced asthma in AIA patients. By comparing D_{limit} and $D_{treshold}$ we are able to explain which patient population is more susceptible to a particular type of NSAID and to evaluate which of the enzymes PGHS1, PGHS2 or LTC_4S might play the central role in aspirin-induced asthma. In our simulations, three different populations of AIA patients are taken into consideration, which differ in expressions, reflecting the activities, of these enzymes; $AIA^{(1)}$: 3-fold lower PGHS1 activity compared to ATA; $AIA^{(2)}$: 5-fold higher LTC_4S activity compared to ATA; $AIA^{(3)}$: 6-fold lower PGHS2 activity compared to ATA. Table 3 shows theoretically determined limiting doses for aspirin ($D_{limit}^{(ASA)}$) and ibuprofen ($D_{limit}^{(IBU)}$) [17] and the intervals or averaged threshold doses from clinical studies [3, 4, 77].

Table 3. Predicted limiting doses for aspirin ($D_{limit}^{(ASA)}$) and ibuprofen ($D_{limit}^{(IBU)}$) in AIA model populations and threshold doses for aspirin ($D_{treshold}^{(ASA)}$) and ibuprofen ($D_{treshold}^{(IBU)}$) for AIA patients [17]

Dose	$AIA^{(1)}$	$AIA^{(2)}$	$AIA^{(3)}$
$D_{limit}^{(ASA)}$ [mg]	455	1025	5150
$D_{limit}^{(IBU)}$ [mg]	16	35	175
$D_{treshold}^{(ASA)}$ [mg]	3 – 600 [4] 325-650 [3]		
$D_{treshold}^{(IBU)}$ [mg]	≅ 400 [77]		

Model results suggest that different AIA model populations show significantly different susceptibilities to aspirin and ibuprofen. Among all three, $AIA^{(1)}$ and partially $AIA^{(2)}$ could be considered as susceptible to aspirin in terms of bronchoconstriction. According to these results, decreased expression of PGHS1 and increased expression of LTC_4S could be considered as the most important factors responsible for the occurrence of bronchoconstriction in AIA patients after aspirin dosing. On the other hand, all three populations could be considered as susceptible to ibuprofen. This is in accordance with the clinical observations in which ibuprofen was recognized as the most frequent initiator for intolerance to NSAIDs [30]. Very high predicted value of $D_{\text{limit}}^{(\text{ASA})}$ in model population $AIA^{(3)}$ indicates that decreased expression of PGHS2 might not be the reason for bronchoconstrictive reactions after challenges with therapeutic doses of aspirin. However, this does not mean that other symptoms of AIA will not occur in this case. In fact, our results suggest the occurrence of chronic symptoms of AIA for this population, since LTC_4 level in the basal state without NSAIDs in this case is several fold higher compared to those in $AIA^{(1)}$ and $AIA^{(2)}$ [16]. The values $D_{\text{limit}}^{(\text{ASA})}$ are much higher than $D_{\text{limit}}^{(\text{IBU})}$. Ibuprofen is thus recognized as a more potent inhibitor of the enzymes PGHS1 and PGHS2 as aspirin. Predicted values of for all three AIA populations are lower than $D_{\text{treshold}}^{(\text{IBU})}$, which is app. 400 mg [77].

It is widely accepted that PGHS1 is a housekeeping enzyme involved in the production of aiPGs [2]. Inflammatory processes in the organism are mainly mediated by piPGs, which are excessively produced by PGHS2 [2]. Usual types of NSAIDs, such as aspirin or ibuprofen, inhibit both enzymes PGHS1 and PGHS2; however, they inhibit PGHS1 more than PGHS2. This is visible from the values of inhibitory constants for PGHS1 (K_{I3}) and for PGHS2 (K_{I1}) for each particular NSAID. For both, aspirin and ibuprofen, K_{I3} is lower than K_{I1}. Since the values of K_I-s reflect the concentration of inhibitor that suppresses the enzyme activity by half (IC50), the lower K_I means the stronger inhibition. Inhibitory action of NSAIDs on both enzymes of the cyclooxygenase pathway reduces the total production of prostaglandins. However, since in the case of aspirin and ibuprofen, PGHS1 is more inhibited than PGHS2, the reduction in aiPGs production is more significant than that in piPGs. The most important aiPG is PGE_2, which regulates the production of LTC_4 through the inhibition of the enzyme 5-LOX. This is believed to increase the production of LTC_4, which finally leads to clinical signs of aspirin-induced asthma in AIA patients. In this context, aspirin-induced asthma could be viewed as a side effect of equal inhibitory actions of aspirin and ibuprofen on both enzymes, however, this does not explain *per se*, why side effects are present only in a part of asthmatic patients. Our model results [16, 17] show and many experiments confirm [11, 51-57] that altered expressions of the key enzymes of AA degradation, PGHS1, PGHS2 and LTC_4S, are essential in occurrence of AIA.

There exist also selective NSAIDs, which inhibit enzyme PGHS2 stronger than PGHS1. These are for example celecoxib, valdecoxib and rofecoxib... Celecoxib is most widely used selective inhibitor in clinical studies [2]. In several studies AIA patients were challenged with a typical therapeutic dose of celecoxib (200 mg) [37, 38] or twice as much [34], and none of the patients reacted. However, there exist rare cases in which AIA patients reacted to these drugs [2]. One reference [39] reports about the person, who did not tolerate 15 mg of celecoxib and 10 mg of aspirin. In what follows, we will compare these clinical data with our theoretically predicted limiting doses for celecoxib ($D_{\text{limit}}^{(\text{CEL})}$) for all three AIA patient populations and will also try to explain this rare case with the model.

Table 4. Theoretically predicted limiting doses for celecoxib for three different AIA patient populations and their comparison with the doses used in provocation tests with AIA patients

Dose	$AIA^{(1)}$	$AIA^{(2)}$	$AIA^{(3)}$
$D_{\text{limit}}^{(\text{CEL})}$ [mg]	115	223	1300
$D_{\text{provocation}}^{(\text{CEL})}$ [mg]	200 mg [37, 38] 400 mg [34]		

Values of presented in Table 4 show that different AIA model populations exhibit different susceptibilities to celecoxib. Population $AIA^{(1)}$ is the most and $AIA^{(3)}$ is the least susceptible to celecoxib. These results are generally in accordance with our previous studies [16, 17], in which we recognized the population $AIA^{(1)}$ as being the most and $AIA^{(3)}$ as being the least susceptible to aspirin and ibuprofen. Since predicted $D_{\text{limit}}^{(\text{CEL})}$ for $AIA^{(3)}$ is higher than doses used in provocation tests [34, 37, 38], population $AIA^{(3)}$ will likely not undergo bronchoconstriction for typical therapeutic doses of celecoxib. For this patient population, bronchoconstriction or symptoms of AIA might occur at higher celecoxib doses than those used in clinical practice. Predicted

$D_{\text{limit}}^{(\text{CEL})}$ for population $\text{AIA}^{(1)}$ is 115 mg and is lower than the reported values [34, 37, 38] and, $D_{\text{limit}}^{(\text{CEL})}$ for $\text{AIA}^{(2)}$, which is 223 mg, falls directly within the reported interval of the doses, used in the provocation tests. The model thus predicts that already typical therapeutic doses of celecoxib might be potentially unsafe for selected AIA populations. It is also interesting how the model can explain a rare case reporting susceptibility of a person to 15 mg dose of celecoxib and 10 mg of aspirin. Our model simulations show that this special case can be explained by approximately 6-fold lower activity of PGHS1 compared to ATA. In comparison to $\text{AIA}^{(1)}$, which is defined by 3-fold lower expression of PGHS1 than ATA, this means additional 2-fold lower expression of PGHS1. In this case, model predicts $D_{\text{limit}}^{(\text{CEL})}=15$ mg and $D_{\text{limit}}^{(\text{ASA})} \cong 10$ mg, as reported [39]. We searched also for other possible theoretical solutions. By taking into account the higher activity of LTC_4S and the lower activity of PGHS2 in the model, other theoretical predictions are possible, but very unlikely. For example, $D_{\text{limit}}^{(\text{CEL})}=15$ mg could be achieved with 40-times and $D_{\text{limit}}^{(\text{ASA})}=10$ mg with 120-times higher activity of LTC_4S. Values for PGHS2, needed for achieving these limiting doses, are of several ranges of magnitude lower than those in ATA. However, in avoidance of misinterpretations of the model results, it is also important to note, that not only PGHS1, PGHS2 and LTC_4S activities are those who contribute to high susceptibilities of AIA patients to NSAIDs compared to ATA, but also the increased number of cysLTR [58] or the decreased number of EP receptors [59] might be the reason for that.

Several researchers proposed different strategies that would enable safe administration of NSAIDs to AIA patients. Such strategies are important for AIA patients with frequent headaches and chronic rheumatic diseases [45]. In these cases, continuous therapy with NSAIDs is required. Since there is strong evidence that increased production of cysLTs plays the most important role in the occurrence of inflammatory reactions in aspirin-induced asthma [2], strategies are mainly focused on the inhibition of the enzyme 5-LOX and the decreases in cysLTs biosynthesis. Typical inhibitors of 5-LOX are native PGE_2, synthetic PGE_2 analogue (nocloprost), synthetic PGE_1 analogue (misoprostol) and the drugs such as zileuton and ABT-761. The basic common idea of all the strategies is to decrease the production of cysLTs by inhibiting 5-LOX after NSAID dosing. In this way, bronchoconstriction and other symptoms of aspirin-induced asthma in AIA patients might be avoided. Several clinical studies report that exogenous PGE_2, administered by inhalation in form of aerosol, has protective effects in asthma induced by NSAIDs [14], allergens [47, 48] or exercise [49] in humans. Inhaled PGE_2 prevents aspirin-induced bronchoconstriction and strongly reduces urinary LTE_4 levels in AIA patients [14]. In another study [42], in which AIA patients were treated with 600 mg of zileuton four times daily, it was shown that zileuton lowers urinary LTE_4 levels, inhibits aspirin-induced bronchoconstriction, diminishes nasal dysfunction and even returns the sense of smell. ABT-761 is another 5-LOX inhibitor that could be used in strategies for safe managing of AIA patients with NSAIDs. This is a novel and potent second-generation 5-LOX inhibitor, which may offer significant improvements in terms of the potency of 5-LOX inhibition and the duration of reduced cysLT biosynthesis as well as in pharmacokinetic properties compared to zileuton [75]. ABT-761 has very slow elimination phase compared to aspirin and ibuprofen, as well as compared to PGE_2 analogue – nocloprost (see Figure 3).

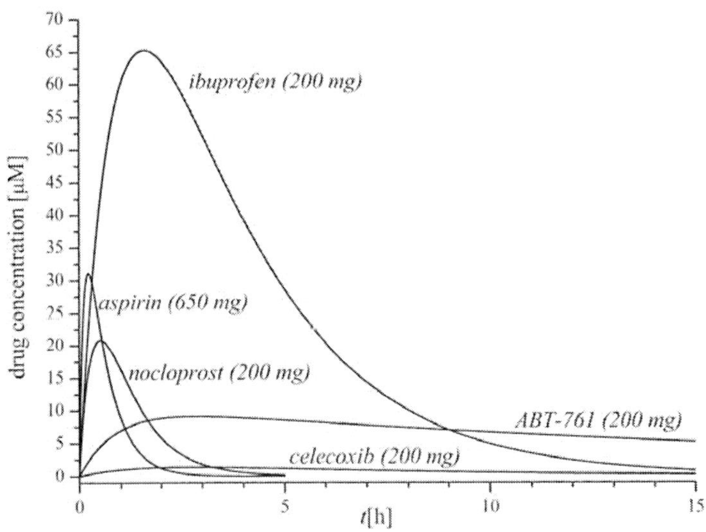

Figure 3. Time courses of plasma drug concentrations for typical doses.

The best strategy for NSAID dosing in combination with ABT-761 is to apply ibuprofen at the time when ABT-761 concentration in blood is maximal; approximately 2.5 hours after ABT-761. This is due to rather slow absorption phase of ABT-761 compared to ibuprofen. In this way, the predicted dose of ABT-761 that should avoid the risk of bronchoconstriction is smaller than in case of taking the drugs at the same time. Predicted doses of ABT-761 in combination to 200 mg in different AIA patient populations are: 510 mg for $AIA^{(1)}$, 700 mg for $AIA^{(2)}$ and 36 mg for $AIA^{(3)}$. The dose of ABT-761 is such, that the relation factor (*Rf*) in our model simulations does not fall below one during the whole period of NSAID action. Although ibuprofen has one of the slowest elimination phases among NSAIDs, there is no need for successive dosing of ABT-761 in combination with ibuprofen. In our recent study [17], we theoretically analyzed another strategy for safe aspirin and ibuprofen dosing to AIA patients; this time in combination with orally stable PGE_2 analogue – nocloprost. The main goal of this study was to determine the exact protocol of PGE_2 analogue dosing in terms of the doses and the times of dosing after ingestion of either aspirin or ibuprofen. In contrast to ABT-761, PGE2 analogue (nocloprost) has much faster absorption and elimination phases so that successive doses after aspirin or ibuprofen are required. The protocol was again such that the value of *Rf* did not drop below one during the whole interval of NSAID presence in plasma. Our model results presented in Table 5 show, that the protocol with PGE2 analogue (nocloprost) is dependent on: i) the population of AIA patients, ii) the differences/similarities of pharmacokinetic properties of NSAID and PGE_2 analogue – nocloprost iii) the dose of NSAID.

Table 5. Protocols for PGE_2 analogue – nocloprost dosing in combination with either 1000 mg of aspirin or 200 mg or 400 mg of ibuprofen in all AIA model populations [17]

Model population	$t_1 = 0$ $D_1^{(PGE_2)}$ [mg]	$t_2 = 2h$ $D_2^{(PGE_2)}$ [mg]	$t_3 = 4h$ $D_3^{(PGE_2)}$ [mg]	$t_4 = 6h$ $D_4^{(PGE_2)}$ [mg]	$t_5 = 8h$ $D_5^{(PGE_2)}$ [mg]
1000 mg aspirin					
$AIA^{(1)}$	15	/	/	/	/
200 mg ibuprofen					
$AIA^{(1)}$	130	100	70	70	/
$AIA^{(2)}$	300	210	150	/	/
$AIA^{(3)}$	30	/	/	/	/
400 mg ibuprofen					
$AIA^{(1)}$	160	120	100	70	60
$AIA^{(2)}$	420	300	210	150	/
$AIA^{(3)}$	160	70	/	/	/

The differences in the predicted protocols for aspirin and ibuprofen as well as for different AIA model patient populations suggest that this protocol, if applied in clinical practice, should certainly be personalized. Partially, this is due to differences in pharmacokinetic properties of aspirin and ibuprofen compared to PGE_2 analogue, and, partially due to differences in susceptibilities between model AIA patient populations. Since absorption and elimination phases of aspirin are similar to those of PGE_2 analogue, the effects of both drugs on AA metabolism appear approximately at the same time. Therefore, already one rather low dose of PGE_2 analogue, applied together with aspirin, is sufficient to prevent bronchoconstriction in all AIA model populations. Since ibuprofen has slower elimination phase compared to PGE_2 analogue, several consecutive doses of PGE_2 analogue are needed to prevent the risk of bronchoconstriction. Also, the doses for ibuprofen are higher, since ibuprofen is stronger inhibitor of both enzymes PGHS1 and PGHS2. Differences also occur between AIA model populations. $AIA^{(2)}$ requires the highest doses and $AIA^{(3)}$ the lowest of PGE_2 analogue – nocloprost.

Conclusion

The mathematical model considers AA degradation *via* lipoxygenase and cyclooxygenase pathways, a production of major eicosanoids as well as interaction of cyclooxygenase pathway with NSAID. In this chapter, our previous versions of the model [16, 17] are upgraded with the involvement of 5-LOX inhibitor. The model incorporates all the main players in AA metabolism and relies on theoretical and experimental biochemical, as well as clinical data in terms of model parameters and variables. Differences between AIA and ATA patients and healthy humans (HH) in expressions of the key enzymes of AA degradation, LTC_4S, PGHS1and PGHS2, are the basis for the definition of our model populations and the proposal for different characterization and subgrouping of AIA patients. In principle, our approach is a systems biology approach in which knowledge from enzyme gene expressions, molecular interactions, pharmacokinetics of drugs and their action on the molecular level as well as implications on the organ level are integrated in the mathematical model, simulations and interpretations of the model results. Furthermore, the model enables simulations of different drugs used in clinical practice: NSAIDs, selective COX inhibitors, exogenous PGE_2 analogues and 5-LOX inhibitors. It contributes to understanding the molecular mechanisms and causal links between the symptoms of AIA, effects of different drugs, their threshold doses, as well as the differences in susceptibilities of individual AIA patients to bronchoconstriction according to different types and doses of NSAIDs. As seen from the results, presented in this chapter and those published elsewhere [16, 17], our model already explains many of them. Furthermore, the additional value of the model is in testing the existing simulations and creating the new ones for different personalized treatment strategies [16, 17].

In addition to the development of the model to such a level that it is applicable in clinical practice for the individualized treatment of AIA patients, the future perspective is also to couple the present model of eicosanoid production with the cell model of bronchial smooth muscle contraction in the view of multiscale modeling [78, 79]. For the purpose of the whole-lung modeling [80], we already developed several whole-cell mathematical models of airway tracheal smooth muscle [81-84], some of them based on the intensive experimental research [81, 83], in which isometric force development in response to cholinergic stimulation is theoretically studied by using computational methods that incorporate biochemical, biophysical and also some anatomical information on cells and tissues. The models introduce an upgrade to the original 4-state latch bridge model, first published by Hai and Murphy [85]. It is upgraded in terms of more sophisticated description of Ca^{2+}-calmodulin (Ca^{2+}-CaM) dependent activation of myosin light chain kinase (MLCK) [86, 87] and its involvement in myosin light chain (MLC) phosphorylation/dephosphorylation process in concordance with myosin light chain phosphatase (MLCP) [81-84]. Based on the measurements of Ca^{2+}-dynamics, performed by our colleges from the Laboratory of respiratory cell physiology at the University of Bordeaux 2 in France [81, 83, 88-91], we are developing and constantly upgrading the models of Ca^{2+} handling in airway smooth muscle cells [90, 92-94]. Therefore, the only missing part, required for the complete integration of the two models (the model of eicosanoid production and the model of bronchial smooth muscle Ca^{2+}-contraction coupling), is probably the link between them. A lot is known about cysLTs binding to cysLTRs and their inhibitors as well as about the effects of both on airway smooth muscle contraction. However, very little is known about the signaling pathways and the molecular mechanisms downstream the cysLTRs. It is hypothesized that in porcine tracheal smooth muscle, for example, LTC_4 might enhance the contraction via the activation of the Rho – Rho-kinase pathway by increasing the Ca^{2+}-responsiveness of the contractile apparatus in a MLC-phosphorylation dependent manner [76]. All this is not far from our very recent experimental and theoretical research, in which we measured the developed force and several other variables. Furthermore, we mathematically modeled the signaling pathways in which Rho-kinase was involved as activator/suppressor of MLCP. Our theoretical results, strongly supported by our measurements [81], evaluate the contribution of the Rho-kinase to the early phase of the Ca^{2+}-dependent airway smooth muscle contraction and give good perspectives for coupling the two models in the view of predictions of the level and the duration of bronchoconstriction after drug dosing.

References

[1] Babu, K.S. and S.S. Salvi, Aspirin and asthma. *Chest*, 2000. 118(5): p. 1470-1476.

[2] Stevenson, D. and A. Szczeklik, Clinical and pathologic perspectives on aspirin sensitivity and asthma. *J Allergy Clin Immunol*, 2006. 118(4): p. 773-786.

[3] Settipane, R.A., et al., Prevalence of Cross-Sensitivity with Acetaminophen in Aspirin-Sensitive Asthmatic Subjects. *Journal of Allergy and Clinical Immunology,* 1995. 96(4): p. 480-485.

[4] Sanchez-Borges, M., NSAID hypersensitivity (respiratory, cutaneous, and generalized anaphylactic symptoms*). Med Clin North Am,* 2010. 94(4): p. 853-864.

[5] Daffern, P.J., et al., Association of urinary leukotriene E4 excretion during aspirin challenges with severity of respiratory responses. *J Allergy Clin Immunol*, 1999. 104(3 Pt 1): p. 559-564.

[6] Micheletto, C., et al., Changes in urinary LTE4 and nasal functions following nasal provocation test with ASA in ASA-tolerant and -intolerant asthmatics. *Respir Med,* 2006. 100(12): p. 2144-2150.

[7] Ferreri, N.R., et al., Release of leukotrienes, prostaglandins, and histamine into nasal secretions of aspirin-sensitive asthmatics during reaction to aspirin. *Am Rev Respir Dis*, 1988. 137(4): p. 847-854.

[8] Sladek, K., et al., Eicosanoids in bronchoalveolar lavage fluid of aspirin-intolerant patients with asthma after aspirin challenge. *Am J Respir Crit Care Med*, 1994. 149(4 Pt 1): p. 940-946.

[9] Settipane, G., Asthma, aspirin intolerance and nasal polyps. N *Engl Reg Allergy Proc*, 1986. 7(1): p. 32-37.

[10] Samter, M. and R.F. Beers, Jr., Concerning the nature of intolerance to aspirin. *J Allergy*, 1967. 40(5): p. 281-293.

[11] Szczeklik, A. and D. Stevenson, Aspirin-induced asthma: advances in pathogenesis and management. *J Allergy Clin Immunol*, 1999. 104(1): p. 5-13.

[12] Vargaftig, B.B. and M. Singer, Leukotrienes mediate murine bronchopulmonary hyperreactivity, inflammation, and part of mucosal metaplasia and tissue injury induced by recombinant murine interleukin-13. *Am J Respir Cell Mol Biol*, 2003. 28(4): p. 410-419.

[13] Gupta, N., M. Gresser, and A. Ford-Hutchinson, Kinetic mechanism of glutathione conjugation to leukotriene A4 by leukotriene C4 synthase. *Biochim Biophys Acta*, 1998. 1391(2): p. 157-68.

[14] Sestini, P., et al., Inhaled PGE2 prevents aspirin-induced bronchoconstriction and urinary LTE4 excretion in aspirin-sensitive asthma. *Am J Respir Crit Care Med*, 1996. 153(2): p. 572-575.

[15] Drazen, J.M., Leukotrienes as mediators of airway obstruction. *Am J Respir Crit Care Med,* 1998. 158(5 Pt 3): p. S193-200.

[16] Dobovisek, A., A. Fajmut, and M. Brumen, Role of expression of prostaglandin synthases 1 and 2 and leukotriene C4 synthase in aspirin-intolerant asthma: a theoretical study. *J Pharmacokinet Pharmacodyn*, 2011. 38(2): p. 261-278.

[17] Dobovisek, A., A. Fajmut, and M. Brumen, Strategy for NSAID administration to aspirin-intolerant asthmatics in combination with PGE2 analogue: a theoretical approach. *Med Biol Eng Comput*, 2012. 50(1): p. 33-42.

[18] Smith, W.L., E.A. Meade, and D.L. Dwitt, Pharmacology of prostaglandin endoperoxide synthase isozymes-1 and-2a. *Annals of the New York Academy of Sciences,* 1994. 714(1): p. 136-142.

[19] Christman, B.W., et al., Prostaglandin E2 limits arachidonic acid availability and inhibits leukotriene B4 synthesis in rat alveolar macrophages by a nonphospholipase A2 mechanism. *J Immunol*, 1993. 151(4): p. 2096-2104.

[20] Harizi, H., et al., Prostaglandins inhibit 5-lipoxygenase-activating protein expression and leukotriene B4 production from dendritic cells via an IL-10-dependent mechanism. *J Immunol*, 2003. 170(1): p. 139-146.

[21] Kay, L., W. Yeo, and P. Peachell, Prostaglandin E2 activates EP2 receptors to inhibit human lung mast cell degranulation. *Br J Pharmacol*, 2006. 147(7): p. 707-713.

[22] Hartney, J.M., et al., Prostaglandin E2 protects lower airways against bronchoconstriction. *Am J Physiol Lung Cell Mol Physiol*, 2006. 290(1): p. L105-113.

[23] Nguyen, M., et al., Receptors and signaling mechanisms required for prostaglandin E2-mediated regulation of mast cell degranulation and IL-6 production. *J Immunol*, 2002. 169(8): p. 4586-4593.

[24] Szczeklik, A. and M. Sanak, The broken balance in aspirin hypersensitivity. *Eur J Pharmacol*, 2006. 533(1-3): p. 145-155.

[25] Maxis, K., et al., The shunt from the cyclooxygenase to lipoxygenase pathway in human osteoarthritic subchondral osteoblasts is linked with a variable expression of the 5-lipoxygenase-activating protein. *Arthritis Res Ther*, 2006. 8(6): p. R181.

[26] Meade, E., W. Smith, and D. DeWitt, Differential inhibition of prostaglandin endoperoxide synthase (cyclooxygenase) isozymes by aspirin and other non-steroidal anti- inflammatory drugs. *J. Biol. Chem.*, 1993. 268(9): p. 6610-6614.

[27] So, O.-Y., et al., The dynamics of prostaglandin H synthases. Studies with prostaglandin H synthase 2 Y355F unmask mechanisms of time-dependent inhibition and allosteric activation. *J Biol Chem*, 1998. 273(10): p. 5801-5807.

[28] Vane, J. and R. Botting, Inflammation and the mechanism of action of anti-inflammatory drugs. *FASEB J*, 1987. 1(2): p. 89-96.

[29] Berges-Gimeno, M.P., R.A. Simon, and D.D. Stevenson, The natural history and clinical characteristics of aspirin-exacerbated respiratory disease. *Ann Allergy Asthma Immunol*, 2002. 89(5): p. 474-478.

[30] Rosado, A., et al., Intolerance to non-steroidal anti inflammatory drugs with respiratory reaction: clinical and diagnostic features. *Alergol Inmunol Clin*, 2000. 15: p. 153-159.

[31] Bianco, S., et al., Efficacy and tolerability of nimesulide in asthmatic patients intolerant to aspirin. *Drugs*, 1993. 46 Suppl 1: p. 115-120.

[32] Kosnik, M., et al., Relative safety of meloxicam in NSAID-intolerant patients. *Allergy*, 1998. 53(12): p. 1231-1233.

[33] Stevenson, D.D. and R.A. Simon, Lack of cross-reactivity between rofecoxib and aspirin in aspirin-sensitive patients with asthma. *J Allergy Clin Immunol*, 2001. 108(1): p. 47-51.

[34] Gyllfors, P., et al., Biochemical and clinical evidence that aspirin-intolerant asthmatic subjects tolerate the cyclooxygenase 2-selective analgetic drug celecoxib. *J Allergy Clin Immunol*, 2003. 111(5): p. 1116-1121.

[35] Martin-Garcia, C., et al., Safety of a cyclooxygenase-2 inhibitor in patients with aspirin-sensitive asthma. *Chest*, 2002. 121(6): p. 1812-1817.

[36] Szczeklik, A., et al., Safety of a specific COX-2 inhibitor in aspirin-induced asthma. *Clin Exp Allergy*, 2001. 31(2): p. 219-225.

[37] Woessner, K.M., R.A. Simon, and D.D. Stevenson, The safety of celecoxib in patients with aspirin-sensitive asthma. *Arthritis Rheum*, 2002. 46(8): p. 2201-2206.

[38] Yoshida, S., et al., Selective cyclo-oxygenase 2 inhibitor in patients with aspirin-induced asthma. *J Allergy Clin Immunol*, 2000. 106(6): p. 1201-1202.

[39] Baldassarre, S., et al., Asthma attacks induced by low doses of celecoxib, aspirin, and acetaminophen. *J Allergy Clin Immunol*, 2006. 117(1): p. 215-217.

[40] Szczeklik, A., Prostaglandin E2 and aspirin-induced asthma. *Lancet*, 1995. 345(8956): p. 1056.

[41] Schafer, D., et al., Dynamics of eicosanoids in peripheral blood cells during bronchial provocation in aspirin-intolerant asthmatics. *Eur Respir J*, 1999. 13(3): p. 638-646.

[42] Dahlen, B., et al., Benefits from adding the 5-lipoxygenase inhibitor zileuton to conventional therapy in aspirin-intolerant asthmatics. *Am J Respir Crit Care Med*, 1998. 157(4 Pt 1): p. 1187-1194.

[43] Rao, N.L., et al., Anti-inflammatory activity of a potent, selective leukotriene A4 hydrolase inhibitor in comparison with the 5-lipoxygenase inhibitor zileuton. *J Pharmacol Exp Ther*, 2007. 321(3): p. 1154-1160.

[44] Wong, S., et al., Pharmacokinetics and pharmacodynamics of single and multiple oral doses of a novel 5-lipoxygenase inhibitor (ABT-761) in healthy volunteers. *Clin Pharmacol Ther*, 1998. 63(3): p. 324-31.

[45] Knowles, S.R., et al., Management options for patients with aspirin and nonsteroidal antiinflammatory drug sensitivity. *The Annals of Pharmacotherapy*, 2007. 41(7): p. 1191-1200.

[46] Schafer, D., et al., Effect of prostaglandin E2 on eicosanoid release by human bronchial biopsy specimens from normal and inflamed mucosa. *Thorax*, 1996. 51(9): p. 919-923.

[47] Hartert, T.V., et al., Prostaglandin E(2) decreases allergen-stimulated release of prostaglandin D(2) in airways of subjects with asthma. *Am J Respir Crit Care Med*, 2000. 162(2 Pt 1): p. 637-640.

[48] Gauvreau, G.M., R.M. Watson, and P.M. O'Byrne, Protective effects of inhaled PGE2 on allergen-induced airway responses and airway inflammation. *Am J Respir Crit Care Med*, 1999. 159(1): p. 31-36.

[49] Melillo, E., et al., Effect of inhaled PGE2 on exercise-induced bronchoconstriction in asthmatic subjects. *Am J Respir Crit Care Med*, 1994. 149(5): p. 1138-1141.

[50] Tuber, U., et al., Pharmacokinetics of nocloprost in human volunteers and its relation to dose. *Eur J Clin Pharmacol*, 1993. 44(5): p. 497-500.

[51] Picado, C., et al., Cyclooxygenase-2 mRNA is downexpressed in nasal polyps from aspirin-sensitive asthmatics. *Am J Respir Crit Care Med*, 1999. 160(1): p. 291-296.

[52] Pujols, L., et al., Dynamics of COX-2 in nasal mucosa and nasal polyps from aspirin-tolerant and aspirin-intolerant patients with asthma. *J Allergy Clin Immunol*, 2004. 114(4): p. 814-819.

[53] Pierzchalska, M., et al., Deficient prostaglandin E2 production by bronchial fibroblasts of asthmatic patients, with special reference to aspirin-induced asthma. *J Allergy Clin Immunol*, 2003. 111(5): p. 1041-1048.

[54] Cowburn, A.S., et al., Overexpression of leukotriene C4 synthase in bronchial biopsies from patients with aspirin-intolerant asthma. *J Clin Invest*, 1998. 101(4): p. 834-846.

[55] Sousa, A., et al., Enhanced expression of cyclo-oxygenase isoenzyme 2 (COX-2) in asthmatic airways and its cellular distribution in aspirin-sensitive asthma. *Thorax*, 1997. 52(11): p. 940-945.

[56] Sanak, M., et al., Enhanced expression of the leukotriene C(4) synthase due to overactive transcription of an allelic variant associated with aspirin-intolerant asthma. *Am J Respir Cell Mol Biol*, 2000. 23(3): p. 290-296.

[57] Sampson, A., et al., Profound overexpression of leukotriene C4 synthase in bronchial biopsies from aspirin-intolerant asthmatic patients. *Int Arch Allergy Immunol*, 1997. 113(1-3): p. 355-357.

[58] Sousa, A.R., et al., Leukotriene-receptor expression on nasal mucosal inflammatory cells in aspirin-sensitive rhinosinusitis. *N Engl J Med*, 2002. 347(19): p. 1493-1499.

[59] Ying, S., et al., Aspirin-sensitive rhinosinusitis is associated with reduced E-prostanoid 2 receptor expression on nasal mucosal inflammatory cells. *J Allergy Clin Immunol*, 2006. 117(2): p. 312-318.

[60] Callan, O.H., O.-Y. So, and D.C. Swinney, The kinetic factors that determine the affinity and selectivity for slow binding inhibition of

human prostaglandin H synthase 1 and 2 by indomethacin and flurbiprofen. *J Biol Chem,* 1996. 271(7): p. 3548-3554.

[61] Gonchar, M., et al., Kinetics of prostanoid synthesis by macrophages is regulated by arachidonic acid sources. *Eur J Biochem*, 1999. 265(2): p. 779-787.

[62] Aharony, D. and R. Stein, Kinetic mechanism of guinea pig neutrophil 5-lipoxygenase. *J Biol Chem*, 1986. 261(25): p. 11512-11519.

[63] Owen, W.F., Jr., et al., Synthesis and release of leukotriene C4 by human eosinophils. *J Immunol*, 1987. 138(2): p. 532-538.

[64] Haeggstrom, J., et al., Guinea-pig liver leukotriene A4 hydrolase. Purification, characterization and structural properties. *Eur J Biochem*, 1988. 174(4): p. 717-724.

[65] Lam, B.K., et al., The mechanism of leukotriene B4 export from human polymorphonuclear leukocytes. *J Biol Chem*, 1990. 265(23): p. 13438-13441.

[66] Meade, E.A., W.L. Smith, and D.L. DeWitt, Differential inhibition of prostaglandin endoperoxide synthase (cyclooxygenase) isozymes by aspirin and other non-steroidal anti-inflammatory drugs. *J Biol Chem*, 1993. 268(9): p. 6610-6614.

[67] Mitchell, J.A., et al., Selectivity of nonsteroidal antiinflammatory drugs as inhibitors of constitutive and inducible cyclooxygenase. *Proc Natl Acad Sci U S A,* 1993. 90(24): p. 11693-11697.

[68] Goltsov, A., et al., In silico screening of nonsteroidal anti-inflammatory drugs and their combined action on prostaglandin H synthase-1. *Pharmaceuticals*, 2010. 3(7): p. 2059-2081.

[69] Noguchi, M., et al., Interfacial kinetic reaction of human 5-lipoxygenase. *Eur J Biochem*, 1994. 222(2): p. 285-292.

[70] Bell, R.L., et al., ABT-761 attenuates bronchoconstriction and pulmonary inflammation in rodents. *J Pharmacol Exp Ther,* 1997. 280(3): p. 1366-1373.

[71] Gupta, N., M.J. Gresser, and A.W. Ford-Hutchinson, Kinetic mechanism of glutathione conjugation to leukotriene A4 by leukotriene C4 synthase. *Biochim Biophys Acta*, 1998. 1391(2): p. 157-168.

[72] Rowland, M., et al., Absorption kinetics of aspirin in man following oral administration of an aqueous solution. *J Pharm Sci*, 1972. 61(3): p. 379-385.

[73] Klueglich, M., et al., Ibuprofen extrudate, a novel, rapidly dissolving ibuprofen formulation: relative bioavailability compared to ibuprofen

lysinate and regular ibuprofen, and food effect on all formulations. *J Clin Pharmacol*, 2005. 45(9): p. 1055-1061.

[74] Paulson, S.K., et al., Pharmacokinetics of celecoxib after oral administration in dogs and humans: effect of food and site of absorption. *J Pharmacol Exp Ther*, 2001. 297(2): p. 638-645.

[75] Wong, S.L., et al., Dose-proportional pharmacokinetics of a new 5-lipoxygenase inhibitor, ABT-761, in healthy volunteers. *Biopharm Drug Dispos,* 1998. 19(3): p. 159-162.

[76] Setoguchi, H., et al., Leukotriene C(4) enhances the contraction of porcine tracheal smooth muscle through the activation of Y-27632, a rho kinase inhibitor, sensitive pathway. *Br J Pharmacol*, 2001. 132(1): p. 11111-8.

[77] Varghese, M. and R.F. Lockey, Aspirin-exacerbated asthma. *Allergy Asthma Clin Immunol*, 2008. 4(2): p. 75-83.

[78] Hunter, P., P. Robbins, and D. Noble, The IUPS human Physiome Project. *Pflugers Arch*, 2002. 445(1): p. 1-9.

[79] Hunter, P.J. and T.K. Borg, Integration from proteins to organs: the Physiome Project. *Nat Rev Mol Cell Biol*, 2003. 4(3): p. 237-243.

[80] Tawhai, M.H., E.A. Hoffman, and C.L. Lin, The lung physiome: merging imaging-based measures with predictive computational models. *Wiley Interdiscip Rev Syst Biol Med*, 2009. 1(1): p. 61-72.

[81] Mbikou, P., et al., Contribution of Rho kinase to the early phase of the calcium-contraction coupling in airway smooth muscle. *Exp Physiol*, 2011. 96(2): p. 240-258.

[82] Fajmut, A. and M. Brumen, MLC-kinase/phosphatase control of Ca2+ signal transduction in airway smooth muscles. *J Theor Biol*, 2008. 252(3): p. 474-481.

[83] Mbikou, P., et al., Theoretical and experimental investigation of calcium-contraction coupling in airway smooth muscle. *Cell Biochem Biophys,* 2006. 46(3): p. 233-252.

[84] Fajmut, A., A. Dobovisek, and M. Brumen, Mathematical modeling of the relation between myosin phosphorylation and stress development in smooth muscles. *J Chem Inf Model,* 2005. 45(6): p. 1610-1615.

[85] Hai, C.M. and R.A. Murphy, Cross-bridge phosphorylation and regulation of latch state in smooth muscle. *Am J Physiol*, 1988. 254(1 Pt 1): p. C99-106.

[86] Fajmut, A., M. Jagodic, and M. Brumen, Mathematical modeling of the myosin light chain kinase activation. *J Chem Inf Model*, 2005. 45(6): p. 1605-9.

[87] Fajmut, A., M. Brumen, and S. Schuster, Theoretical model of the interactions between Ca2+, calmodulin and myosin light chain kinase. *FEBS Lett,* 2005. 579(20): p. 4361-4366.

[88] Belouchi, N.E., et al., Effect of chronic hypoxia on calcium signalling in airway smooth muscle cells. *Eur Respir J,* 1999. 14(1): p. 74-79.

[89] Belouchi, N.E., et al., Interaction of extracellular albumin and intravenous anaesthetics, etomidate and propofol, on calcium signalling in rat airway smooth muscle cells. *Fundam Clin Pharmacol*, 2000. 14(4): p. 395-400.

[90] Marhl, M., et al., Importance of cell variability for calcium signaling in rat airway myocytes. *Biophys Chem*, 2010. 148(1-3): p. 42-50.

[91] Roux, E., et al., Calcium signaling in airway smooth muscle cells is altered by in vitro exposure to the aldehyde acrolein. Am J Respir Cell Mol Biol, 1998. 19(3): p. 437-444.

[92] Brumen, M., et al., Mathematical modelling of Ca2+ oscillations in airway smooth muscle cells. Journal of Biological Physics, 2005. 31(3): p. 515-524.

[93] Roux, E. and M. Marhl, Role of sarcoplasmic reticulum and mitochondria in Ca2+ removal in airway myocytes. Biophys J, 2004. 86(4): p. 2583-2595.

[94] Haberichter, T., et al., The influence of different InsP(3) receptor isoforms on Ca(2+) signaling in tracheal smooth muscle cells. Bioelectrochemistry, 2002. 57(2): p. 129-138.

In: Asthma: Causes, Complications and Treatment ISBN: 978-1-62257-447-6
Editors: A. H. Bislimi and L. C. Tolka

Chapter II

The Role of Neuroimmune and Psychological Systems in the Pathophysiology of Bronchial Asthma

***Ervin Ç. Mingomataj*[1,2,*] *and Alketa H. Bakiri*[3]**
[1]"Mother Theresa" School of Medicine, Department of Allergology & Clinical Immunology, Tirana, Albania
[2]University of Tirana, Nursing Faculty, Department of Preclinical Disciplines, Albania
[3]Albanian University, Faculty of Stomatology, Department of Preclinical Disciplines, Tirana, Albania

Abstract

Bronchial asthma (BA) is a pathologic disorder, characterized by reversible obstruction, bronchial inflammation and hyperreactivity, bronchial mucus secretion, systemic and local eosinophilia, as well as increased IgE level in serum. Apart from immune mechanisms, several researches point out that asthmatics could be distinguished by a psychological profile described as halfway between patients with mood

* Corresponding address: Ervin Ç. Mingomataj, Rruga Myslym Shyri, P. 47, Apt. 15, Tirana – Albania. E-mail: allergology@gmx.de.

disorders or anxiety and general population. In addition, the BA or allergic airway inflammation in experimental animals are associated with induction of pro-inflammatory neurotrophins or neuropeptides such as nerve growth factor (NGF), tachykinin peptides substance P (SP) and neurokinin A in bronchoalveolar lavage or nodose sensory neurons innervating lower airways. Using retrograde neuronal tracing technique in combination with double-labeling immunohistochemistry, the allergic sensitization of these animals has been associated with an induction of tachykinin predominantly in airway-specific large-sized (myelinated) jugular–nodose ganglia neurons. Similar changes with respect to neurotrophin / tachykinin labeling are reported in the limbic system after stress-related experiments, while the increased seric level of mentioned neuropeptides is associated with anxious or depressive disorders. These findings suggest that allergen sensitization / challenge (as well as stressful events) may lead to the *de novo* induction of tachykinins in neurons probably via epigenetic mechanisms, putting neuropsychological system of affected subject in a defensive alarming state. It could be concluded that besides the use of bronchodilators and anti-inflammatory medications, the pharmacologic depletion of neuroimmune mechanisms and the consideration of the BA as a psychosomatic and depressive-associated disorder ("bronchial hysteria") may improve the therapeutic approaches in the future.

Keywords: Bronchial asthma, neuroimmune mechanisms, tachykinins, psychosomatic disorders

The world is changing at faster pace than mankind adaption!

1. Definition of Bronchial Asthma

Bronchial asthma (BA) is characterized by a chronic inflammatory process of the airways, which in general, includes variable airflow obstruction, airway hyperresponsiveness, immunoglobulin (Ig)E-response to aeroallergens, mucus production, eosinophilic infiltration, and epithelial denudation [1-6]. The inflammatory process is followed by healing, the end result of which is an altered structure referred to as airway remodeling [1]. This pathology is considered a T helper (Th)2-type disorder frequently associated with atopy, eosinophilia and allergic comorbidities [3, 7, 8]. However, the Th1 cell-associated cytokine interferon (IFN)-γ, absence of IgE response and airway neutrophilia has been implicated in some severe phenotypes of BA [3, 9,

10]. Gene array studies in allergised mice demonstrated that mast cell expression of receptor IFN-γR contributed to the development of receptor FcεRIγ-dependent and some FcεRIγ-independent features of disease. These features include the airway hyperresponsiveness, neutrophilic and eosinophilic inflammation, airway remodeling, and lung expression of several cytokines, chemokines, and markers of an alternatively activated macrophage response [3, 9]. Targeting the components of the disease with selective therapies has been disappointing and most therapy still relies on bronchodilators and corticosteroids rather than treating underlying disease mechanisms [8]. However, involvement of small airways causing air trapping appears to be crucial in making BA refractory to classic treatment [9].

2. Bronchial Asthma Is not only an Immune Disorder

The lack of a strong correlation between the clinical severity and the expression of immuno-inflammatory mechanisms in the allergic BA has lead to the suggestion that other factors independent to the activation of immune mechanisms are capable to induce symptoms of this pathology. Regarding development of respiratory allergies, an important topic of studies in recent decades has been the neurogenic inflammation [2]. Thus, elevated neurotrophin concentrations have been shown in nasal and bronchoalveolar lavage (BAL) fluids as well as in the sera of patients with allergic rhinitis and BA. According to some reports, concentration of nerve growth factor (NGF) correlated with disease severity, airways hyperreactivity, and levels of mediators released from eosinophils [2]. Due to the release of cationic proteins, oxygen species, and cytokines after degranulation, eosinophils contribute to tissue damage and can influence airway hyperresponsiveness in BA. Moreover, several studies have reported about a high incidence of well structured psychiatric disorders in asthmatic patients, while other authors have pointed out just a psychological behavior characterized by anxious and depressive traits [11-13]. The aim of this review is to elucidate the dimensions of direct and indirect neuro-psychological mechanisms contributing to development of the BA.

3. Neuroimmune Mechanisms in Development of Bronchial Asthma

The neurotrophins NGF, brain-derived neurotrophic factor (BDNF), neurotrophin-3 (NT-3) and NT-4 play a pivotal role in the development of the nervous system [14]. Despite their well-known effects on neurons, elevated neurotrophin concentrations have been observed under pathological conditions in sera of patients with inflammatory disorders. Patients with BA feature both airway inflammation and abnormal airway reactivity to many unspecific stimuli, referred to as airway hyperresponsiveness, which is, at least partly, neuronally controlled [14]. Neurotrophins can mediate such effects due to receptor stimulation. Thus, the presence of neurotrophins and the neurotrophin receptors p75 (p75NTR), tyrosine kinase A (TrkA), TrkB and TrkC have been described not only in neuronal cells but also in several immune cells [14]. Meanwhile, the stimulation of neurotrophin receptors is associated with synthesis and release of tachykinins [15]. The tachykinins are members of the family of closely related neuropeptides comprising substance P (SP), neurokinin A (NKA) and NKB, etc. These peptides are encoded by the PPT-A gene and are widely but selectively expressed throughout the central and peripheral nervous system, where their functions were first identified as neurotransmitters [16]. Tachykinins are involved in the pathogenesis of pain, inflammatory bowel disease, rheumatoid arthritis and airway inflammatory diseases such as BA [15, 17-19].

In fact, airway nerves have the capacity to control airway functions via nervous reflexes and through neuropeptides, such as tachykinins. The responsible neuronal mechanisms play a key role in the initiation and modulation of airway hyperresponsiveness and inflammation [15, 20-22]. Thus, the tachykinin peptides, SP, NKA, and the related neuropeptide calcitonin gene-related peptide (CGRP), are known to have potent pro-inflammatory effects in the airways. In experimental trials, they can be released from sensory nerve endings mainly originating from the jugular ganglia to the guinea-pig and rat airways [15, 23-26]. In addition, studies in mice demonstrated that treatment with a dual neurokinin receptor NK-1/NK-2 antagonist partly prevents allergic airway inflammation in a transgenic mouse model [15]. The NK-1 and NK-2 are respective receptors for tachykinins SP and NKA (see Figure 1 - adapted from [27]) [15].

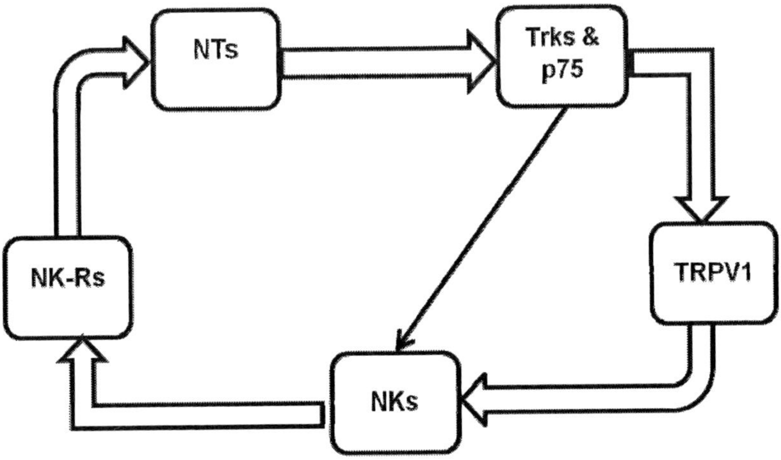

Legend: NTs – neurotrophins, Trks & p75 – Tyrosinekinases and p75 NT-receptors, NKs – neurokinins (SP, NKA), NK-Rs – neurokinin receptors (NK-1, NK-2).

Figure 1. The cycle of neurotrophin-related pathways in the development of bronchial asthma.

Besides the sensory origin from the jugular and nodose ganglia, the lower airways are also innervated by thoracic spinal afferents which originate from dorsal root ganglia (DRG) neurons [26, 28-30]. This innervation has the capacity to release a variety of mediators such as SP/NKA and CGRP in response to a broad range of stimuli including capsaicin, bradykinin, hyperosmolar saline, tobacco smoke and cold dry air [28, 31-33]. The extent of the observed morphological co-localization of TrkA and transient receptor potential cation channel subfamily V member 1 (TRPV1) with SP, suggests that the DRG pathway may also have some effects on the magnitude of neurogenic inflammation in airway diseases such as BA [28]. However, the physiological importance of DRG neurons in airway inflammation remains to be determined. In this respect, future functional studies may reveal the full extend by which the DRG pathway contributes to neuronal processes underlying airway inflammation [28].

Nevertheless, tachykinins such as SP/NKA and CGRP can be released to the site of inflammation by axonal transport and by activation of the TRPV1 receptor [15, 31, 33–35]. In the airways released from afferent nerve terminals, SP acts on NK1-receptors and mediates neurogenic inflammation. This process can be described as a complex response consisting of increased vascular permeability, plasma extravasation, glandular secretion, pro-inflammatory cell influx and pulmonary vascular remodeling [15, 34–36]. In an experimental study conducted by Dinh et al. in mice, tachykinins were extendedly expressed in small airway specific sensory neurons of ganglia jugularum nodosum with diameters smaller than 20 mm under normal conditions [15]. This finding suggests that expression of tachykinins was found in airway-specific sensory neurons, previously identified as capsaicin-sensitive and TRPV1 positive sensory neurons [37]. Similar results reported that tachykinergic neurons innervating the airways of guinea-pigs were also C-fiber profiles [24, 38]. Interestingly, the induction of *de novo* tachykinin synthesis was predominantly found in large-diameter airway-specific neurons in mice with allergic airway inflammation [15]. The inflammation was confirmed by an increase in the number of leucocytes and eosinophils recovered from BAL fluids in these animals [24, 25]. The induction of tachykinins in vagal sensory neurons has already been described even in guinea-pig airways by allergen and NGF treatment [38, 39] and murine airways by injection of NGF into the airways [15, 28]. Previously, the induction of tachykinins was found in neurons with neurofilament-immunoreactivities (also described as fast-conducting Aδ-fibers) [15, 38]. In the study conducted by Dinh et al., the induction of tachykinins was found in large-diameter neurons that may express neurofilament protein and probably belong to the cell bodies of Aδ-fibers [15]. Such patho-physiological changes are also described in the trigeminal neurons of mice after intranasal application of the NGF [22]. The NGF caused neuronal changes by induction of SP expression in trigeminal neurons innervating the nasal mucosa of the mouse. Similarly to the SP induction by allergen, the highest level of SP expression in trigeminal neurons was found at the time-point 24h after NGF injection. After 36h, the numbers of neurons with SP have been rapidly reduced and returned back to the basal level 3 days after NGF injection [22-25, 40]. According to the same study, NGF induced the SP-expression in trigeminal neurons that mostly belonged to the neurofilament-positive subpopulation. These neurons are mechanically sensitive and belong to the fast-conducting neuronal Aδ-fibers [38]. In contrast to the lower airway vagal neurons, SP induction was also found in a small numbers of nasal-specific neurons that were non-reactive for neurofilament immunoreactivity [22].

Clinically, the sensorial airway innervation is of potential interest as contributory factors in the pathogenesis of chronic upper airway diseases such as allergic rhinitis [22, 41]. The respective nerves may cause rhinorrhea and congestion, which are major symptoms of this disorder [40, 42]. Nasal-specific sensory nerves are known to be derived from trigeminal neurons and have the capacity to synthesize a variety of mediators such as tachykinins SP and NKA under normal and pathological conditions [22, 43-45]. They were predominantly located to a region close to the division of the ophthalmic and maxillary nerves as reported by a previous study [22, 40, 43]. Centrally, SP can evoke nasonasal reflex mechanism, partly to protect the upper and lower airways [43, 46]. Dinh et al. reported that all SP-positive sensory neurons also expressed TRPV1. This extent of presently examined total co-localization of SP and TRPV1 may indicate a functional role of TRPV1 in SP biosynthesis and release [43]. In this context, using a TRPV1 antagonist termed capsazepin, it was shown that SP release from sensory nerves can be efficiently inhibited [43, 47]. The present neurochemical findings support the hypothesis, that the SP-pathway may be partly TRPV1-dependent [43]. The extent of SP and TRPV1 co-localization in nasal sensory neurons suggests that, following a peripheral activation of the TRPV1 receptor on SP afferents, there may be a triggering of SP-mediated phenomena such as neurogenic inflammation [43].

Taken together, these findings indicate that the heterogeneity of neuronal subpopulations concerning their peptide profiles may have different functions in nasal reflex activity and neurogenic airway inflammation [22, 43, 48]. With respect to the SP induction mostly in neurofilament-positive, myelinated Aδ-fibers neurons of the upper and lower airways during allergic or NGF stimulation, it could be suggested that an acute inflammatory process could lead to the local hyperresponsiveness toward various specific or unspecific stimuli [15, 22, 38]. This might be a possible scenario, because the sensorial airways innervation can switch to an alarming state under the effect of different inducers. Under such circumstances, each stimulus can trigger a defensive reflex in the sensorial network of airways. In our opinion, the neuronal impulse spreads quickly along airways, if more and more Aδ-fibers are switched-on with respect to SP-synthesis [49]. The pathological consequence of this switch could be the induction of bronchial or nasal hyperreactivity, associated with occurrence of relative neuro-inflammatory symptoms.

4. Experimental Models of Stress induce Similar Effects in the Bronchial Mucosa

In the recent years is demonstrated that BA-related immune and neuronal mediators can be induced in stress situations [50, 51]. In a murine model, sound stress enhances allergic airway inflammation rather identified by leukocyte numbers and eotaxin level than by Th2-cytokines level in BAL fluids [51]. In the same murine stress model or after SP-application was revealed an increased percentage of TNF-α-positive T cells in lymph nodes [52]. In addition, sound stress alone or in combination with OVA-sensitization and challenge induces a similar SP-synthesis in vagal sensory neurons related to bronchial mucosa [52]. Thus, stress significantly increased PPT-A mRNA expression in lung tissue from OVA-sensitized and -challenged animals, and immune cells were identified as an additional source of SP in the lung by immunohistochemistry [51]. The significant increase of leukocyte number in BAL fluids and the enhanced airway reactivity in stressed and OVA-sensitized/challenged mice were blocked by treatment of animals with a NK-1 receptor antagonist [53]. These data provide further evidence for a stress-mediating neuro-immunological pathway that, putatively via SP, is able to influence the composition of immune cells in different compartments of allergic airway inflammation [52].

5. Bronchial Asthma Is Associated with Clinical Anxious-depressive Symptoms

The relationship between BA and a particular psychological profile has been studied for many years [11, 54-56]. Several studies have shown a high incidence of well structured psychiatric disorders in asthmatic patients, while other authors have pointed out just a psychological behavior characterized by anxious and depressive traits [11, 13]. Some authors share the opinion that mentioned subjects can be distinguished by a psychological profile described as a halfway between patients with anxiety, mood disorders and the general population [11, 57].

Such associations between a somatic disease and psychological disorders are reported even in patients with rheumatoid arthritis, cardiovascular diseases, recurrent abdominal pains, diabetes mellitus, etc [13, 58, 59]. Nevertheless, the association of BA with psychological disorders is better argued. A clinical study conducted in outpatient subjects demonstrated that potential depressive symptoms are more evident among asthmatics than patients with diabetes, gastro-hepathologic disorders and healthy subjects [12, 13]. The obtained data suggested that both being chronic and the specificity of asthmatic disease are probable inducing factors with regard to depressive symptoms. Moreover, this survey demonstrated that severe asthmatics developed more frequently depressive symptoms [13]. Similarly to this study, Chetta et al have reported that asthmatic subjects with severe disease developed more frequently hypochondriasis, psychological disturbances such as agoraphobia or panic disorders, and poor perception of breathlessness [60]. In addition, patients with "brittle" asthma have greater psychiatric morbidity than those with less severe asthma [60, 61]. These findings agree with a survey conducted by Brown et al., which demonstrated that among patients of moderate to severe BA treated community, health facilities may have high rates of often untreated mood and anxiety disorders [62]. Higher rates of psychiatric disorders by asthmatics in comparison to healthy subjects are also reported by Campbell and Mrazek, which has been linked to more severe disease, increased length of stay in hospital, and increased use of steroid medication [13, 61]. In addition, Ten Brinke et al. reported that presence of psychopathologic disorder in patients with severe BA increases odds ratios for frequent visits to general physicians, frequent emergency units, frequent exacerbations, and frequent hospitalizations [63]. This indicates that the morbidity and costs of BA might be related to the level of psychological dysfunction in patients with severe asthma rather than to asthma severity per se [13, 63]. Meanwhile, Kilpeläinen et al. reported that stressful life events promote the manifestation of BA and atopic diseases, indicating the evidence of stress-induced alteration in immune-mediated diseases [13, 64].

Even if the presence of a chronic disease like BA in the family can be a reason of stress increase, further experimental studies have demonstrated an interaction between inflammatory cells in the lungs, production of IgE, induction of bronchial hyperreactivity or local eosinophilic inflammation, and nervous system [65, 66]. This complex interaction, explains partially the relation between allergic airway disease and psychological stress [65, 66]. Thus, the nervous stimulation can promote mast cell degranulation due to axon reflexes [13, 67]. Moreover, stressful events and atopic diseases like BA are shown to induce neurotrophin synthesis and release in BAL fluids and plasma [68-72]. Some studies in mice have demonstrated that stress enhances airway reactivity and airway inflammation in experimental models [50-52, 65]. In this context, such neuromediators like SP or other neurokinins are involved in the same manner in peripheral sensory fibers of the airways after allergic sensitization or permanent stress in experimental studies in mice [15, 51].

Regarding the central nervous system, these mediators are distributed in some limbic regions like hippocampus or amygdale [73, 74]. These neuronal structures are involved in potentiation of defensive rage behavior or neuronal firing in response to stress [73, 74]. Notably, the specific role of neuromediators in the BA was described only after the finding of an increased NGF-level in all subjects immediately before parachute jumping, while the same observation was described only in an asthmatic subject who was participating in the control group [13, 68]. Recently, the experimental treatment with neurotrophin and neurokinin antagonists demonstrated not only anti-depressive effects, but also inhibitory effects regarding airway hyperreactivity [51, 73, 74]. Meanwhile, the under-expression of these neurotransmitters or their receptors is associated with inhibition of the expected response to stressful events, or may lead to the mutilation behaviors like in schizophrenia [13, 73, 75]. Similarly to neuroimmune mediators, the pro-allergic immune profile may also explain the association between these pathologies. In this respect, Pavon et al. reported about a Th2 response in such psychological disorders, which are characteristic of allergic pathologies [76, 77].

In summary, these findings suggest that asthmatic patients might need a special psychological check-up to clarify the presence of the depressive disorders and the introduction of respective therapies if it were reasonable [13]. Despite the objective limitations, the time and resource investment employed in gathering such data seems to be an effective as well as efficient way of proceeding, which could beneficial for a better fitted treatment of asthmatic patients in the future [11].

6. Bronchial Asthma as Psychosomatic Disease

The origin of concept "illness" is not based on the pathology but in the suffering, which can be realized due to nervous system and psyche [78-80]. Because of frequent anxious-depressive symptoms among asthmatics, some authors share the idea that BA is really a psychosomatic disorder [62, 64, 79-82]. Siefert, in its opinion, pretends that either the pathology is psychosomatic or it does not exist at all [83, 84]. Logically, the question would be: Are the depressive psychoses detected among the asthmatic subjects, consequences of continuous suffering or consistent part of the pathology? According to the psychosomatologist von Weizsäcker, it exists for the humans the possibility that "either drama of their life can be played on the psychosocial scene or on the somatic one" [85]. When the "personal" on the first scene is tired, the same spectacle could go on the next scene. The content should be not changed; only the costumography represents differences [78, 85]. As a psychosomatic disorder, the BA could be a bio-psychosocial crisis or a "making's suppression", because the pathology should be a disharmony expression of an interrupted composition or an unfulfilled life's motive [85-88]. Self the patients experience the psychosocial dimension of the illness as a personal failure [78, 81]. In other words, the attack of bronchial obstruction could be not considered only bronchial epilepsy but also an expression of "bronchial hysteria" [89]. Once more, these concepts suggest that asthmatic patients might need a special psychological check-up to clarify the presence of the depressive disorders and the introduction of respective therapies if it were reasonable [78].

7. Are Neuronal Mechanisms Involved in the Bronchial Asthma Quite Harmful or rather Inadequate Defenses?

As previously mentioned, airway inflammatory symptoms during BA are mediated through various neurotrophins and their respective receptors [14, 15]. The activation of neurotrophinic receptors induces synthesis of tachykinins such SP and NKA [90-92]. Thus, it is reported about a correlation between the level of mentioned mediators in the BAL or in the lower airways with inflammation level and clinical symptomatology observed in asthmatics or experimental models of the BA [71, 91-93].

Meanwhile, the induction of mentioned neurotrophins promotes an increased survival rate not only for structures within the neuronal system, but also for various kinds of cells in contact with bronchial lumen and noxious stimuli [90-93]. In contrast to other cellular subpopulations of bronchial structures, it emerges an epithelial denudation during the bronchial inflammation (assumed generally to be caused by contact to harmful environmental stimuli) [90, 94]. This effect is associated with potentiation of bronchial hyperresponsiveness, which is mediated by sensorial subepithelial neuronal fibers [90, 91, 95]. The induction of this process could be explained by the fact that potentiation of neurotrophin synthesis within the epithelial cells is associated with an evidence of low levels for relative receptors [90-92, 95]. In other words, the pattern of epithelial response contrasts to the various resident or emigrated cellular subpopulations in the bronchial tissue, which show both neurotrophin and neurotrophin receptor induction [91, 92, 95]. Due to absence of neurotrophin receptors, the bronchial epithelia could be not protected by survival effect of neurotrophins such as NGF, indicating that epithelial-originating neurotrophins can induce only parakrine surviving effects [90-92, 95, 96].

Reflecting on the above-mentioned findings, it might be supposed that epithelial integrity could not be affected only by noxious effect of environmental factors, such as allergens or unspecific stimuli as generally assumed [90]. The loss of neurotrophinic receptors such as TrkA, p75, etc on the epithelial cells may interrupt the neurotrophin-mediated surviving effect, indicating that depletion of this stimulus could be a strategic action of organism to provide bronchial hyperresponsiveness [90]. This effect can be occurred because the sensorial fibers will be more closely to the bronchial lumen after epithelia denudation. Furthermore, the epithelia-synthesized neurotrophins may potentiate also the epithelial destruction due to increase of eosinophil survival rate [90, 97]. In addition, the hyperplasic effect of SP and its receptor NK-1 on the goblet cells contrast with its destructive effect, which is shown on the epithelia of experimentally sensitized mice [98]. All these facts may indicate that inducing the epithelial denudation, asthmatic organism could provide the reduction of contact to harmful stimuli due to consequent bronchial obstruction, trying therefore to provide also a successive suffering relief [90].

The development of BA could be also associated with environmental conditions of modern life, especially the increased life's rhythm and expectations. The allergic respiratory diseases were quite rare at the beginning of last century but their prevalence in industrialized countries has now risen to true epidemic proportions [99-101]. Thus, data from several sources indicate worldwide prevalence increases of BA or allergic rhinitis over the last 30-40 years, especially in English-speaking countries [102, 103]. Although the presence of affected relatives is associated with an increased risk of atopic diseases, recent data suggest that much of the increase in the BA-prevalence is occurring in subjects without a significant genetic predisposition [99, 104]. Thus, described data from MAS cohort study conducted in German children at 5 years of age have shown in a majority of cases that asthmatic subpopulation has originated from non-atopic parents, indicating for the environmental impact on the atopy rising trend [99, 105, 106]. Because this prevalence increase happened relatively in a short period of time, the role of populations' genomic transformation is assumed to be quite limited [101, 103]. Moreover, after the 1950s there was a gradient even between former East and West

Germany regarding the prevalence of atopic diseases, despite the population was genetically the same [101, 107]. Therefore, the almost of epidemiologic studies have pointed out the influence of different environmental risk factors on the rising trend of atopic diseases [99].

Besides the influence of other environmental factors, the atopy rising trend can be associated with affronting of many difficulties in the accomplishment of life expectations, because of unstoppable acceleration of everyday life [99, 105, 108]. For instance, the most characteristic feature of mankind is the tendency to transform the environment in a very short period of time, thus it does not have a fixed and unchanging environment [109]. This period is too short to allow biologic or social adaptation to these changes [99, 109]. Not only the world but also the world perception is changing at a faster pace than mankind-self could be adapted. Consequently, it could be concluded that the chosen environment is unhealthy; therefore certain individuals cannot be adapted to it [109]. If somebody cannot adapt to his environment (and in the case of human beings environment means even a social environment, a certain social structure, institutions, moral-, technical-, etc. standards), it can be often said that he is diseased, but in some cases it can just as rightly be said that the environment is unreasonable [109].

In context of accelerated urbanization, the globalization and high tech information had led to the higher life expectations compared to the former period of times when the world was more isolated. Thus, the much higher (sometimes dizzy) life rhythm and disillusions because of non-fulfillment of own expectations may lead more frequently to disappointments and depressive symptoms as well as to induction of allergic disorders [99, 108]. This scenario may be possible because the same neurological or immunologic mechanisms are similarly regulated in both disorders, which are frequently associated with each other [11, 13, 64, 99]. In other words, similarly to allergic subjects, patients who represent major depressive disorder show a Th2 cytokine profile, whereas mediators of neurogenic inflammation such as the NGF and SP are shown to be overregulated in allergic inflammatory response, stress and depressive diseases [23, 51, 65, 68, 71, 73, 74, 76, 99, 110]. Maybe immigrants (arrived from rural areas or developing countries during last decades), experience this situation relatively late in their lifespan or at least more "violently", and therefore, they are less adapted against these additional challenges [99]. Consequently, their problems can be reflected on the difficult relationships with each-other in their own family or social environment, and on the exacerbating of the immunologic and neuro-psychological disorder.

Reflecting about all the presented facts, it could be suggested that accelerated transformations of the environment and lifestyle as well as the simultaneous non-fulfillment of life expectations (alias the changing world) might be the risk mega-factor for the development of atopic diseases [99]. In other words, maybe this is not per se a risk factor of atopic diseases; rather its components act as risk factors because of inefficient adaptation after short-time exposure toward them for certain subpopulations. If the components of modern environment such as improved hygiene, air pollution, and western lifestyle were part of former traditional life (whereas the components of traditional environment such as anthroposophy were part of actual modern life), the anthroposophy were an expected risk factor for atopic diseases [99]. In the circumstances of the changing world, the prevalence of allergic diseases might be in correlation with respective transformation rhythms.

Despite the influence for a short period of time, it could be not excluded that certain environmental factors may switch the expression of target genes even after exposure cessation in a heritable manner without directly altering the genome, defined as epigenetic mechanisms [111-113]. There is increasing evidence pointing to the influence of prenatal and early life exposures on the development of allergic disease [114]. In particular, a growing body of literature supports the theory that transient environmental pressures can have permanent effects on gene regulation and expression through epigenetic mechanisms [99, 114]. Histone modifications have been associated with degree of bronchial hyperresponsiveness and corticosteroid resistance in BA [111-114]. Epigenetic mechanisms can operate independently in various cell types, such as in human T cells, etc [114]. Meanwhile, murine studies have revealed that a maternal diet rich in methyl donors can enhance susceptibility to allergic inflammation in the offspring, mediated through increased DNA methylation [114]. Additional studies have also implicated epigenetically modified dendritic cells in the transmission of allergic risk from mothers to offspring. However, further human studies are necessary to explore these mechanisms and assess future clinical applicability [114]. Similarly to BA and allergy, Yehuda et al. reported increased prevalence of posttraumatic stress disorder by babies whose pregnant mothers were exposed to the World Trade Center attacks or in adult offspring of Holocaust survivors [99, 115]. Therefore, to elicit the impact of environmental factors on human genome function even after exposure to a risk factor in a short period of time, actually it might be necessary to conduct approaches about the exposure to environmental indoor and outdoor pollutions such as tobacco smoke or diesel exhausts in newborn experimental animals and successively it should be investigated about the immune response, etc after allergenic exposure in their later lifespan or by their offspring [99, 116, 117].

Taken together, the BA could be not only a pathologic development, but also an inadequate attempt to adapt against different stressful conditions [81]. It seems that the activation of neuroimmune and psychological mechanisms is associated with informative signalization abilities mediated by neurotrophin-related pathways, especially expressed in sensorial centers such as spinal, jugular-nodose or trigeminal ganglia, as well as in hippocampus and other consciousness-associated constituent parts of limbic system [27, 28, 53, 118-120]. In addition, these mediators are described in peripheral tissues such as mucosa, inflammatory cells, or in peripheral neuronal fibers [23, 27, 74, 118, 121-123]. On the other hand, the induction of neurokinins and the relative receptors under stimulation of neurotrophins like NGF during inflammatory disorders could be explained with an identification of harmful stimuli [27]. This effect can assure the release of the inflammatory response (including pathologic symptoms such as pain, edema, erythema, or hyperreactivity), which in effect should be considered as a complex of protective mechanisms to escape from the situation [27, 124]. Moreover, the induction of mentioned neurokinins can induce again the increase of neurotrophins, leading to the potentiation of survival rates for various cellular populations [125-127].

These findings may indicate that, independently to the somatic or psychic nature of the disease, the informative language with regards to presupposed harmful stimuli seems to be the same. This is true as long as the difference consists only in the associated brain areas, in which the stimuli are projected [27, 120]. In fact, the informative mediators possess rather detectorial than meaning properties, because the information is produced due to consciousness, while neuronal fibers and mucosa alone are not conscious [120]. During diseases that are associated with increased neurotrophin levels such as allergy, stressful events or depression, the affected subjects can be informed about exposition to real or imaginary dangers, as long as in the reality perceptions are only hypotheses about the environment [27, 53, 92, 120, 128-130]. This opinion could be based on the facts that inflammatory disorders such as the allergy and BA are associated with noxious contact between antigen and organism, while depressive and anxious psychoses are associated with violation of mental and emotional integrity (because of persistent suffering or persistent alert), independently to the fact if stimuli is real or not [27]. The BA is not really mistake, but rather wisdom of the body, because the suffering is not only suffered, but also it will be needed and wanted [81, 131]. In other words, pathologic symptoms are not only signs of disorder, but also body attempts to correct it [27, 88]. While the illness is to can, the sufferings can be defenses [81, 132].

Conclusion

Generally, the BA is considered an immuno-inflammatory disorder of lower airways, but immune alterations do not always relay with development of pathology [2]. Apart from immune mechanisms, many published researches point out that asthmatics seem to be distinguished by a psychological profile described as halfway between patients with mood disorders or anxiety and general population [11-13, 60, 64]. In addition, the BA or allergic airway inflammation in the experimental models may enhance pro-inflammatory neurotrophins or tachykinins such as NGF, BDNF, SP and NKA in BAL fluids or nodose sensory neurons innervating lower airways [14, 15, 22, 27, 28, 43, 122]. Using retrograde neuronal tracing technique in combination with double-labeling immuno-histochemistry, the allergic sensitization of experimental animals has been associated with a tachykinin induction, predominantly detected in airway-specific large-sized (myelinated) jugular–nodose ganglia neurons [15, 22]. Similar changes with respect to neurotrophin / tachykinin labeling are reported in the limbic system after stress-related experiments, while an increased seric level of mentioned neuropeptides is associated with anxious or depressive disorders [13, 69-72]. These findings support the idea that allergen sensitization / challenge may lead to the *de novo* tachykinin-synthesis in the respective neurons probably via epigenetic mechanisms, putting neuropsychological system of affected subject in an alarming state. These alterations can induce the bronchial hyperreactivity and other inflammatory symptoms, suggesting that neuro-psychological mechanisms play a decisive role in the development of the BA. In other words, it should be the switch-on timing of these mechanisms that play a determining role in the occurrence of clinical symptoms and not only the activation of immune mechanisms. This agrees with the fact that the concentration of some allergic mediators such as specific IgE or Th2-cytokines is increased even in normal subjects, while a neuro-psychological or "identity" crisis may trigger the bronchial or psychological disturbances ("the bronchial hysteria") even in subjects who show normal immune mediator concentrations [13].

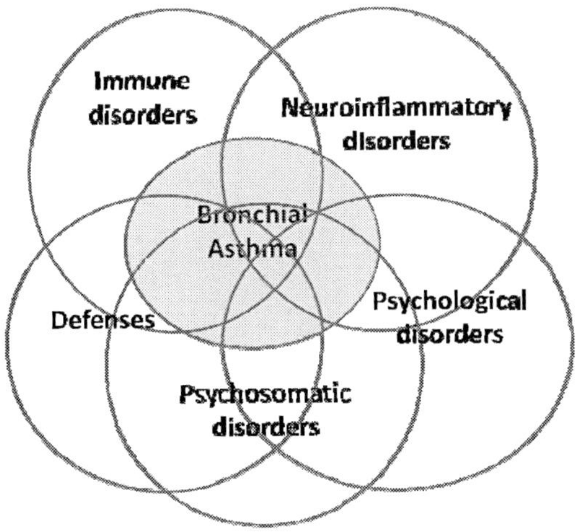

Bronchial asthma can be included in diverse patho-physiological interfering classifications

Figure 2. Clinical dimensions of bronchial asthma.

Taken together, these mechanisms may also indicate that the response against psychological and antigenic "stresses" could be expressed in the same "language" [27]. The induction of SP, NGF, specific IgE, etc might be only a consecutive response against different kinds of harmful stimuli. The trophic function of these neurotransmitters is in the same time a defense and surviving stimulation for the threatened organism [13, 27]. While the patient may experience such stressful situations as a personal breakdown, the consequent development of BA or depression might be simply the same disease expressed in different forms (see Figure 2) [81, 85]. It could be not excluded that besides the traditional use of bronchodilators and anti-inflammatory medications, the pharmacologic depletion of neuroimmune mechanisms and the consideration of the BA as a psychosomatic and depressive-associated disorder (therefore a "bronchial hysteria") may improve the therapeutic approaches in the future [13].

References

[1] Vignola, AM; Gagliardo, R; Siena, A; Chiappara, G; Bonsignore, MR; Bousquet, J; Bonsignore, G. Airway remodeling in the pathogenesis of asthma. *Curr Aller Asthma Rep* 2001, 1, 108-15.

[2] Nassenstein, C; Braun, A; Nockher, WA; Renz, H. Neurotrophin effects on eosinophils in allergic inflammation. *Curr Aller Asthma Rep* 2005, 5, 204-11.

[3] Yu, M; Eckhart, MR; Morgan, AA; Mukai, K; Butte, AJ; Tsai, M; Galli, SJ. Identification of an IFN-γ/mast cell axis in a mouse model of chronic asthma. *J Clin Invest* 2011, 121, 3133-43.

[4] Platts-Mills, TA; Woodfolk, JA. Allergens and their role in the allergic immune response. *Immunol Rev* 2011, 242, 51-68.

[5] Ozdemir, C. Monoclonal antibodiesin allergy; current applications and promising trials. *Recent Pat Inflamm Allergy Drug Discov* 2009, 3, 201-10.

[6] Buc, M; Dzurilla, M; Vrlik, M; Bucova, M. Immunopathogenesis of bronchial asthma. *Arch Immunol Ther Exp* (Warsz) 2009, 57, 331-44.

[7] Holgate, ST. Pathophysiology of asthma: What has our understanding taught us about new therapeutic approaches? *J Aller Clin Immunol* 2011, 128, 495-505.

[8] Holgate, ST; Arshad, HS; Roberts, GC; Howarth, PH; Thurner, P; Davies, DE. A new look at the pathogenesis of asthma. *Clin Sci* (Lond) 2009, 118, 439-50.

[9] Louis, R. Severe asthma: how can we differentiate phenotypes? *Swiss Med Wkly* 2009, 139, 274-7.

[10] Holt, PG; Strickland, DH; Bosco, A; Jahnsen, FL. Pathogenic mechanisms of allergic inflammation: atopic asthma as a paradigm. *Adv Immunol* 2009, 104, 51-113.

[11] Centanni, S; di Marco, F; Castagna, F; Boveri, B; Casanova, F; Piazzini, A. Psychological issues in the treatment of asthmatic patients. *Respir Med* 2000, 94, 742-9.

[12]. Mingomataj, EÇ; Xhixha, F; Muka, L; Duni, A; Gjata, E. Asthmatic patients complain more often about eventual depressive disorders than patients suffering from different chronic digestive pathologies. *Aller & Clin Immunol Int* 2005, (Suppl. 1 - WAO/EAACI Congress – Abstracts Book), P. 247.

[13] Mingomataj, EÇ; Xhixha F; Muka, L; Duni, A; Bakiri, A; Gjata, E; Dinh, QT. [Asthmatics complain more often about eventual depressive disorders than patients with different chronic digestive pathologies]. *Curr Med Nursing Care* (Tirana) 2011, 7, 14-8. [in Albanian]

[14] Nassenstein, C; Kerzel, S; Braun, A. Neurotrophins and neurotrophin receptors in allergic asthma. *Prog Brain Res* 2004, 146, 347-67.

[15] Dinh, QT; Mingomataj, E; Quarcoo, D; Groneberg, DA; Witt, C; Klapp, BF; Braun, A; Fischer, A. Airway allergic inflammation induces tachykinin peptides expression in vagal sensory neurons innervating mouse airways. *Clin Exp Allergy* 2005, 35, 820-5.
[16] Springer, J; McGregor, GP; Fink, L; Fischer, A. Alternative splicing in single cells dissected from complex tissues: separate expression of preprotachykinin A mRNA splice variants in sensory neurons. *J Neurochem* 2003, 85, 882–8.
[17] Mantyh, CR; Vigna, SR; Bollinger, RR; Mantyh, PW; Maggio, JE; Pappas, TN. Differential expression of substance P receptors in patients with Crohn's disease and ulcerative colitis. *Gastroenterol* 1995, 109, 850–60.
[18] Bulling, DG; Kelly, D; Bond, S; McQueen, DS; Seckl, JR. Adjuvant-induced joint inflammation causes very rapid transcription of beta-preprotachykinin and alpha-CGRP genes in innervating sensory ganglia. *J Neurochem* 2001, 77, 372–82.
[19] Barnes, PJ; Chung, KF; Page, CP. Inflammatory mediators of asthma: an update. *Pharmacol Rev* 1998, 50, 515–96.
[20] Barnes, PJ. Asthma as an axon reflex. *Lancet* 1986, 1, 242–5.
[21] Carr, MJ; Undem, BJ. Pharmacology of vagal afferent nerve activity in guinea pig airways. *Pulm Pharmacol Ther* 2003, 16, 45–52.
[22] Mingomataj, E; Dinh, QT; Groneberg, D; Wu, S; Feleszko, W; Schmeck, B; Joachim, R; Noga, O; Nagel, S; Klapp, BF; Fischer, A. Trigeminal nasal-specific neurons respond to nerve growth factor with substance-P biosynthesis. *Clin Exp Allergy* 2008, 38, 1203-11.
[23] Fischer, A; McGregor, GP; Saria, A; Philippin, B; Kummer, W. Induction of tachykinin gene and peptide expression in guinea pig nodose primary afferent neurons by allergic airway inflammation. *J Clin Invest* 1996, 98, 2284–91.
[24] Myers, AC; Kajekar, R; Undem, BJ. Allergic inflammation-induced neuropeptide production in rapidly adapting afferent nerves in guinea pig airways. *Am J Physiol Lung Cell Mol Physiol* 2002, 282, 775–81.
[25] Undem, BJ; Hunter, DD; Liu, M; Haak-Frendscho, M; Oakragly, A; Fischer, A. Allergen-induced sensory neuroplasticity in airways. *Int Arch Aller Immunol* 1999, 118, 150–3.
[26] Springall, DR; Cadieux, A; Oliveira, H; Su, H; Royston, D; Polak, JM. Retrograde tracing shows that CGRP-immunoreactive nerves of rat trachea and lung originate from vagal and dorsal root ganglia. *J Auton Nerv Syst* 1987, 20, 155–66.

[27] Mingomataj, EÇ. The pleiotropism of nerve growth factor sensorial pathway: supplemental growth stimuli could be required during danger signalization like as surviving proclaim. *Irn J Med Hypotheses Ideas* 2008, 2, 16.

[28] Dinh, QT; Groneberg, DA; Peiser, C; Mingomataj, E; Joachim, RA; Witt, C; Arck, PC; Klapp, BF; Fischer, A. Substance P expression in TRPV1 and trkA-positive dorsal root ganglion neurons innervating the mouse lung. *Respir Physiol Neurobiol* 2004, 144, 15-24.

[29] Kummer, W; Fischer, A; Kurkowski, R; Heym, C. The sensory and sympathetic innervation of guinea-pig lung and trachea as studied by retrograde neuronal tracing and double-labelling immunohistochemistry. *Neuroscience* 1992, 49, 715–37.

[30] Lundberg, JM; Brodin, E; Saria, A. Effects and distribution of vagal capsaicin-sensitive substance P neurons with special reference to the trachea and lungs. *Acta Physiol Scand* 1983, 119, 243–52.

[31] Fischer, A; Folkerts, G; Geppetti, P; Groneberg, DA. Mediators of asthma: nitric oxide. *Pulm Pharmacol Ther* 2002, 15, 73–81.

[32] Groneberg, DA; Fischer, A. Endogenous opioids as mediators of asthma. *Pulm Pharmacol Ther* 2001, 14, 383–89.

[33] Groneberg, DA; Springer, J; Fischer, A. Vasoactive intestinal polypeptide as mediator of asthma. *Pulm Pharmacol Ther* 2001, 14, 391–401.

[34] Springer, J; Geppetti, P; Fischer, A; Groneberg, DA. Calcitonin gene-related peptide as inflammatory mediator. *Pulm Pharmacol Ther* 2003, 16, 121–30.

[35] Caterina, MJ; Schumacher, MA; Tominaga, M; Rosen, TA; Levine, JD; Julius, D. The capsaicin receptor: a heat-activated ion channel in the pain pathway. *Nature* 1997, 389, 816–24.

[36] Springer, J; Fischer, A. Substance P-induced pulmonary vascular remodelling in precision cut lung slices. *Eur Respir J* 2003, 22, 596–601.

[37] Kollarik, M; Dinh, QT; Fischer, A; Undem, BJ. Capsaicin-sensitive and -insensitive vagal bronchopulmonary C-fibres in the mouse. *J Physiol* 2003, 551, 869–79.

[38] Hunter, DD; Myers, AC; Undem, BJ. Nerve growth factor-induced phenotypic switch in guinea pig airway sensory neurons. *Am J Respir Crit Care Med* 2000, 161, 1985–90.

[39] De Vries, A; Dessing, MC; Engels, F; Henricks, PA; Nijkamp, FP. Nerve growth factor induces a neurokinin-1 receptor-mediated airway

hyperresponsiveness in guinea pigs. *Am J Respir Crit Care Med* 1999, 159, 1541–4.

[40] Hunter, DD; Dey, RD. Identification and neuropeptide content of trigeminal neurons innervating the rat nasal epithelium. *Neuroscience* 1998, 83, 591–9.

[41] Anggard, A. Basic mechanisms in autonomic nervous responses in specific and nonspecific nasal hyperreactivity. *Acta Otolaryngol* 1993, 113, 394–6.

[42] Baraniuk, JN; Kaliner, M. Neuropeptides and nasal secretion. *Am J Physiol* 1991, 261, L223–35.

[43] Dinh, QT; Groneberg, DA; Mingomataj, E; Peiser, C; Heppt, W; Dinh, S; Arck, PC; Klapp BF; Fischer, A. Expression of substance P and vanilloid receptor (VR1) in trigeminal sensory neuron projecting to the mouse nasal mucosa. *Neuropeptides* 2003, 37, 245-50.

[44] Lundblad, L. Protective reflexes and vascular effects in the nasal mucosa elicited by activation of capsaicin-sensitive substance P-immunoreactive trigeminal neurons. *Acta Physiol Scand* 1984, 529(Suppl.), 1–42.

[45] Geppetti, P; Fusco, BM; Marabini, S; Maggi,CA; Fanciullacci, M; Sicuteri, F. Secretion, pain and sneezing induced by the application of capsaicin to the nasal mucosa in man. *Br J Pharmacol* 1988, 93, 509–14.

[46] Lacroix, JS; Potter, EK. Nasonasal reflex mechanisms in anaesthetized dogs. *Acta Otolaryngol* 1999, 119, 249–56.

[47] McVey, DC; Vigna, SR. The capsaicin VR1 receptor mediates substance P release in toxin A-induced enteritis in rats. *Peptides* 2001, 22, 1439–46.

[48] Taylor-Clark, TE; Kollarik, M; McGlashan, DW Jr; Undem, BJ. Nasal sensory nerve populations responding to histamine and capsaicin. *J Aller Clin Immunol* 2005, 116, 1282–8.

[49] Ricco, MM; Kummer, W; Biglari, B; Meyers, AC; Undem, BJ. Interganglionic segregation of distinct vagal afferent fibre phenotypes in guinea–pig airways. *J Physiol* (London) 1996, 496, 52–30.

[50] Joachim, RA; Sagach, V; Quarcoo, D; Dinh, QT; Arck, PC; Klapp, BF. Effect of stress on eotaxin and expression of adhesion molecules in a murine model of allergic airway inflammation. *J Neuroimmunol* 2007, 182, 55-62.

[51] Joachim, RA; Cifuentes, LB; Sagach, V; Quarcoo, D; Hagen, E; Arck, PC; Fischer, A; Klapp, BF; Dinh, QT. Stress induces substance P in

vagal sensory neurons innervating the mouse airways. *Clin Exp Allergy* 2006, 36, 1001-10.

[52] Joachim, RA; Sagach, V; Quarcoo, D; Dinh, QT; Arck, PC; Klapp, BF. Upregulation of tumor necrosis factor-alpha by stress and substance p in a murine model of allergic airway inflammation. *Neuroimmune modulation* 2006, 13, 43-50.

[53] Joachim, RA; Sagach, V; Quarcoo, D; Dinh, QT; Arck, PC; Klapp, BF. Neurokinin-1 receptor mediates stress-exacerbated allergic airway inflammation and airway hyperresponsiveness in mice. *Psychosom Med* 2004, 66, 564-71.

[54] Thompson, WL; Thompson, TL. Psychiatric aspects of asthma in adults. *Adv Psychosom Med* 1985, 14, 33-47.

[55] Spector, F; Luparello, TJ. Response of asthmatics to metacholine and suggestion. *Am Rev Respir Dis* 1976, 113, 43-50.

[56] Staudenmayer, H; Kinsman, RA; Dirks, JF; Spector, SL; Wangaard, C. Medical outcome in asthmatic patients: effects on airways hyperreactivity and symptom-focused anxiety. *Psychosom Med* 1979, 41, 109-18.

[57] Belloch, A; Perpina, M; Paredes, P; Gimenez, A; Compte, L; Banos, R. Bronchial asthma and personality dimension: a multifaceted association. *J Asthma* 1994, 31, 161-70.

[58] Strine, TW; Ford, ES; Balluz, L; Chapman, DP. Risk behaviors and health-related quality of life among adults with asthma. *Chest* 2004, 126, 1849–54.

[59] Chapman, DP; Perry, GS; Strine, TW. The vital link between chronic disease and depressive disorders. *Prev Chron Dis: Pub Health Res Pract Policy* 2005, 2, 1–10.

[60] Chetta, A; Gerra, G; Foresi, A; Zaimovic, A; del Donno, M; Chittolini, B; Malorgio, R; Castagnaro, A; Olivieri, D. Personality profiles and breathlessness perception in outpatients with different gradings of asthma. *Am J Respir Crit Care Med* 1998, 157, 116-22.

[61] Garden, GMF; Ayres, JG. Psychiatric and social aspects of brittle asthma. *Thorax* 1993, 48, 501-5.

[62] Brown, ES; Khan, DA; Mahadi, S. Psychiatric diagnoses in inner city outpatients with moderate to severe asthma. *Int J Psychiatry Med* 2000, 30, 319-27.

[63] Ten Brinke, A; Ouwerkerk, ME; Zwinderman, AH; Spinhoven, P; Bel, EH. Psychopathology in patients with severe asthma is associated with

increased health care utilization. *Am J Respir Crit Care Med* 2001, 163, 1093-6.

[64] Kilpeläinen, M; Koskenvuo, M; Helenius, H; Terho, EO. Stressful life events promote the manifestation of asthma and atopic diseases. *Clin Exp Allergy* 2002, 32, 256-63.

[65] Joachim, RA; Quarcoo, D; Arck, PC; Herz, U; Renz, H; Klapp, BF. Stress enhances airway reactivity and airway inflammation in an animal model of allergic bronchial asthma. *Psychosom Med* 2003, 65, 811-5.

[66] Persoons, JHA; Berkenbosch, F; Schornagel, K; Thepen, T; Kraal, G. Increased specific IgE production in lungs after the introduction of acute stress in rats. *J Aller Clin Immunol* 1995, 95, 765-70.

[67] Bienenstock, J; MacQueen, G; Sestini, P; Marshall, JS; Stead, RH; Perdue, MH. Mast cell/nerve interactions in vitro and in vivo. *Am Rev Respir Dis* 1991, 143, 55-8.

[68] Aloe, L; Bracci-Laudiero, L; Alleva, L; Lambiase, E; Micera, A; Tirassa, P. Emotional stress induced by parachute jumping enhances blood nerve growth factor levels and the distribution of the nerve growth factor receptors in lymphocytes. *Proc Natl Acad Sci USA* 1994, 91, 10440-4.

[69] Alleva, E; Petruzzi, S; Cirulli, F; Aloe, L. NGF regulatory role in stress and coping of rodents and humans. *Pharmacol Biochem Behav* 1996, 54, 65-72.

[70] Alleva, E; Aloe, L; Cirulli, F; della Setta, D; Tirassa, P. Serum NGF levels increase during lactation and following maternal aggression in mice. *Physiol Behav* 1996, 3, 461-6.

[71] Bonini, S; Lambiase, A; Bonini, S; Angelucci, F; Magrini, L; Manni, L; Aloe, L. Circulating nerve growth factor levels are increased in humans with allergic diseases and asthma. *Proc Natl Acad Sci USA* 1996, 93, 10955-60.

[72] Alleva, E; Santucci, D. Psychosocial vs. "physical" stress situations in rodents and humans: role of neurotrophins. *Physiol Behav* 2001, 73, 313-20.

[73] Bersani, G; Iannitelli, A; Fiore, M; Angelucci, F; Aloe, L. Data and hypotheses on the role of nerve growth factor and other neurotrophins in psychiatric disorders. *Med Hypotheses* 2000, 55, 199-207.

[74] Stout, SC; Owens, MJ; Nemeroff, CB. Neurokinin-1 receptor antagonists as potential antidepressants. *Annu Rev Pharmacol Toxicol* 2001, 41, 877-906.

[75] Indo, Y. Molecular basis of congenital insensivity to pain with anhidrosis (CIPA): mutations and polymorphism in Trk A (NTRK1) gene encoding the receptor tyrosine kinase for nerve growth factor. *Human Mutation* 2001, 18, 462–71.

[76] Pavon, L; Sandoval–Lopez, G; Eugenia Hernandez, M; Loria, F; Estrada, I; Perez, M; Moreno, J; Avila, U; Leff, P; Anton, B; Heinze, G. Th2 cytokine response in major depressive disorder patients before treatment. *J Neuroimmunol* 2006, 172, 156-65.

[77] Mingomataj, EÇ; Xhixha, F; Gjata, E. Helminths can protect themselves against rejection inhibiting hostile respiratory allergy symptoms. *Allergy* 2006, 61, 400–6.

[78] Mingomataj, E. [Bronchial asthma as illness and its existential meaning]. *Curr Med Nursing Care* (Tirana) 2006, 2, 6-13. [in Albanian]

[79] Cluley, S; Cochrane, GM. Psychological disorder in asthma is associated with poor control and poor adherence to inhaled steroids. *Respir Med* 2001, 95, 37–9.

[80] Kielholz, P; Beck, D. Vegetative Untersuchungen und Theorie der Erschöpfungs-depression. *Praxis* 1962, 51, 39.

[81] Overbeck, G. Krankheit als Anpassung. Der sozio–psychosomatische Zirkel. *Suhrkamp Verlag*, Frankfurt /M. 1984.

[82] Mrazek, DA. Psychiatric complications of pediatric asthma. *Ann Allergy* 1992, 69, 285– 93.

[83] Siefert, H. Sigmund Freund, Georg Groddeck und die psychosomatische Medizin. *Prax Psychother Psychosom* 1979, 24, 63.

[84] Egger, J. Gibt es „psychosomatische" Krankheiten? In: Egger J (Hrsg.) Psychologie in der Medizin. *Medizinische Psychologie, Psychotherapie, Psychosomatik.* Wien, Wiener Universitätsverlag WUV 1993, 106–23.

[85] Danzer, G. Medizinkritik: Der Streit um den kranken Menschen. In: Pieringer W, und Ebner F (Hrsg): *Zur Philosophie der Medizin.* Springer Verlag, Wien 2000.

[86] Engel, GL, Schmale, AH. Eine Psychoanalytische Theorie der somatischen Störung. *Psyche* 1969, 23, 241.

[87] Egger, WJ. Die evolutionäre Erkenntnistheorie und der biopsychosoziale Krankheitsbegriff in der Medizin. In: Pieringer W, und Ebner F (Hrsg): *Zur Philosophie der Medizin.* Springer Verlag, Wien 2000.

[88] Pieringer, W. Theorien und Methoden der Humanmedizin. In: Pieringer W, und Ebner F (Hrsg): *Zur Philosophie der Medizin.* Springer Verlag, Wien 2000.

[89] Hoang, BX. Bronchial epilepsy of broncho-pulmonary hyper-excitability as a model of asthma pathogenesis. *Med Hypotheses* 2006, 67, 1042-51.

[90] Mingomataj, EÇ. The absence of supplemental induction of neurotrophin receptors on the bronchial epithelia during bronchial asthma may lead to the epithelial denudation. *Biosci Hypotheses* 2008, 1, 112-4.

[91] Kerzel, S; Päth, G; Nockher, WA; Quarcoo, D; Raap, U; Groneberg, DA; Dinh, QT; Fischer, A; Braun, A; Renz, H. Pan neurotrophin receptor p75 contributes to neuronal hyperreactivity and airway inflammation in a murine model of asthma. *Am J Respir Cell Mol Biol* 2003, 28, 170-8.

[92] De Vries, A; Engels, F; Henricks, PA; Leusink-Muis, T; McGregor, GP; Braun, A; Groneberg, DA; Dessing, MC; Nijkamp, FP; Fischer, A. Airway hyper-responsiveness in allergic asthma in guinea-pigs is mediated by nerve growth factor via the induction of substance P: a potential role for trkA. *Clin Exp Allergy* 2006, 36, 1192-200.

[93] Levi-Montalcini, R. The nerve growth factor 35 years later. *Science* 1987, 237, 1154–62.

[94] Barbato, A; Turato, G; Baraldo, S; Bazzan, E; Calabrese, F; Panizzolo, C; Zanin, ME; Zuin, R; Maestrelli, P; Fabbri, LM; Saetta, M. Epithelial damage and angiogenesis in the airways of children with asthma. *Am J Respir Crit Care Med* 2006, 174, 975-81.

[95] Frossard, N; Freund, V; Advenier, C. Nerve growth factor and its receptors in asthma and inflammation. *Eur J Pharmacol* 2004, 500, 453-65.

[96] Zampieri, N; Chao, MV. Mechanisms of neurotrophin receptor signalling. *Biochem Soc Transactions* 2006, 34, 607-11.

[97] Mingomataj, EÇ. Eosinophil-induced prognosis improvement of solid tumors could be enabled by their vesicle-mediated barrier permeability induction. *Med Hypotheses* 2008, 70, 582-4.

[98] Springer, J; Groneberg, DA; Dinh, QT; Quarcoo, D; Hamelmann, E; Braun-Dullaeus, RC; Geppetti, P; Anker, SD; Fischer, A. Neurokinin-1 receptor activation induces the reactive oxygen species and epithelial damage in airway allergic inflammation. *Clin Exp Allergy* 2007, 37, 1788-97.

[99] Mingomataj, E. The changing world as principal reason for atopy rising trend. *Intern J Asthma Allergol Immunol* 2007, 5, 2.

[100] Burney, PGJ; Luczynska, C; Chinn, S; Jarvis, D. The European Community Respiratory Health Survey. *Eur Respir J* 1994, 7, 954-60.

[101] Bjorksten, B; Dumitrascu, D; Foucard, T; Khetsuriani, N; Khaitov, R; Leja, M; Lis, G; Pekkanen, J; Priftanji, A; Riikjarv, MA. Prevalence of childhood asthma, rhinitis and eczema in Scandinavia and Eastern Europe. *Eur Respir J* 1998, 12, 432-7.

[102] Sly, RM. Changing prevalence of allergic rhinitis and asthma. *Ann Allergy Asthma Immunol* 1999, 82, 233-48.

[103] Davies, RJ; Rusznak, C; Devalia, JL. Why is allergy increasing? – Environmental factors. *Clin Exp Allergy* 1998, 28, 8-14.

[104] Christie, GL; McDougall, CM; Helms, PJ. Is the increase in asthma prevalence occurring in children without a family history of atopy? *Scott Med J* 1998, 43, 180-2.

[105] Mingomataj, EÇ; Xhixha, F; Gjata, E; Hyso, E; Qirko, E. Prevalence of a family history of atopic disease among 3 generations of atopic respiratory patients in Tirana, Albania. *J Invest Allergol Clin Immunol* 2008, 18, 190-3.

[106] Wahn, U. What drives the allergic march? Allergy 2000, 55, 591-9.

[107] Wichmann, HE. Possible explanation for the different trends of asthma and allergy in East and West Germany. *Clin Exp Allergy* 1996, 26, 621-3.

[108] Ring, J. [Allergology since Clemens von Pirquet 1906-2006]. *Allergo J* 2006, 15, 334-7. [in German]

[109] Kovacs, J. The concept of health and disease. *Med Health Care Philosophy* 1998, 1, 31-9.

[110] Black, PH. Stress and the inflammatory response: A review of neurogenic inflammation. *Brain Behav Immunity* 2002, 16, 622-53.

[111] Wolffe, AP; Matzke, MA. Epigenetics: regulation through repression. *Science* 1999, 286, 481-6.

[112] Levenson, JM; Sweatt, JD. Epigenetic mechanisms in memory formation. *Nat Rev Neurosci* 2005, 6, 108-18.

[113] Sutherland, JE; Costa, M. Epigenetics and the environment. *Ann N Y Acad Sci* 2003, 983, 151-60.

[114] North, ML; Ellis, AK. The role of epigenetics in the developmental origins of allergic disease. *Ann Aller Asthma Immunol* 2011, 106, 355-61.

[115] Yehuda, R; Engel, SM; Brand, SR; Seckl, J; Marcus, SM; Berkowitz, GS. Transgenerational effects of posttraumatic stress disorder in babies

of mothers exposed to the World Trade Center attacks during pregnancy. *Clin Endocrinol Metab* 2005, 90, 4115-8.

[116] Schumacher, A; Petronis, A. Epigenetics of complex diseases: from general theory to laboratory experiments. *Curr Top Microbiol Immunol* 2006, 310, 81-115.

[117] Mager, J; Bartolomei, MS. Strategies for dissecting epigenetic mechanisms in the mouse. *Nat Genet* 2005, 37, 1194-200.

[118] Facer, P; Casula, MA; Smith, GD; Benham, CD; Chessell, IP; Bountra, C; Sinisi, M; Birch, R; Anand, P. Differential expression of the capsaicin receptor TRPV1 and related novel receptors TRPV3, TRPV4, and TRPM8 in normal human tissues and changes in traumatic and diabetic neuropathy. *BMC Neurol* 2007, 7, 11.

[119] Cirulli, F; Capone, F; Bonsignore, LT; Aloe, L; Alleva, E. Early behavioural enrichment in the form of handling renders mouse pups unresponsive to anxiolytic drugs and increases NGF levels in the hippocampus. *Behavior Brain Research* 2007, 178, 208-15.

[120] Roth, G. Das Gehirn und seine Wirklichkeit. Kognitive Neurobiologie und ihre philosophischen Konsequenzen. *Suhrkamp Verlag*, Frankfurt / M 1996.

[121] Hoyle, GW; Graham, RM; Finkelstein, JB; Kim–Phuong, TN; Gozal D; Friedman, M. Hyperinnervation of the airways in transgenic mice overexpressing nerve growth factor. *Am J Respir Cell Mol Biol* 1998, 18, 149–57.

[122] Nassenstein, C; Mayer, S; Braun, A; Lommatzsch, M; Renz, H; Luttmann, W; Virchow, JC. Die mögliche Bedeutung der Neurotrophine in der Pathogenese des allergischen Asthmas. *Allergologie* 2001, 24, 408–18.

[123] Diogenes, A; Akopian, AN; Hargreaves, KM. NGF up-regulates TRPA1: implications for orofacial pain. *J Dent Research* 2007, 86, 550-5.

[124] Frith, CD. The neurocognitive neuropsychology of schizophrenia. Earlbeaum L. Hove: Hillsdale, 1992.

[125] Dekkers, W. Health and illness: From an analytical to a hermeneutical approach. *Med Health Care Philosophy* 1999, 2, 315–8.

[126] Svenaeus, F. The hermeneutics of medicine and the phenomenology of health: Steps towards a philosophy of medical practice. *Linköping University*, Linköping 1999.

[127] Williams, CG. Pleiotropy, natural selection, and the evolution of senescence. *Evolution* 1957, 11, 398–411.

[128] Kimata, H. Effect of exposure to volatile organic compounds on plasma levels of neuropeptides, nerve growth factor and histamine in patients with self-reported multiple chemical sensitivity. *Int J Hygiene Environ Health* 2004, 207, 159-63.

[129] Angelucci, F; Mathe, AA; Aloe, L. Neurotrophic factors and CNS disorders: findings in rodent models of depression and schizophrenia. *Progr Brain Research* 2004, 146, 151-65.

[130] Faure, J; Uys, JD; Marais, L; Stein, DJ; Daniels, WM. Early maternal separation alters the response to traumatization: resulting in increased levels of hippocampal neurotrophic factors. *Metabol Brain Diseases* 2007, 22, 183-95.

[131] Von Weizsäcker, V. Körpergeschehen und Neurose. *Klett*, Stuttgart 1947.

[132] Williams, GW; Nesse, RM. The down of Darwinian medicine. *Quarterly Review of Biology* 1991, 66, 1–22.

In: Asthma: Causes, Complications and Treatment ISBN: 978-1-62257-447-6
Editors: A. H. Bislimi and L. C. Tolka

Chapter III

Special Considerations of Asthma in Older Adults

***Pooja Oza*[1] *and Sharmilee M. Nyenhuis*[2,*]**
[1]Department of Pediatrics, University of Illinois at Chicago, US
[2] Section of Pulmonary, Critical Care, Sleep and Allergy, Department of Medicine, University of Illinois at Chicago, IL, US

Abstract

Asthma is a complex disorder characterized by variable and recurring symptoms of airflow obstruction, bronchial hyperresponsiveness, and underlying inflammation. Although asthma is commonly thought of as a disease of children and young adults, a significant percentage (4-13%) of the older adult (>65 years old) population in the United States is affected and carry a higher rate of morbidity and mortality from the disease. Despite this relatively large prevalence, asthma is often underdiagnosed and undertreated in older adults. The diagnosis of asthma in older adults is challenging due to comorbid conditions and the broad differential diagnosis of other diseases that can produce symptoms similar to asthma. Moreover, older adults have diminished lung and immune function, which can further complicate the disease. A comprehensive assessment that focuses on these issues is necessary to improve the diagnosis and guide therapeutic interventions in

* Corresponding author: Sharmilee M. Nyenhuis 840 S. Wood St. MC 719/920N-CSB Chicago, IL 60612 Email: snyenhui@uic.edu. Fax: 312-996-4665. Phone: 312-413-1655.

older asthmatics. Finally, there are complexities in the management of asthma that are unique to older adults, including the adverse effects of medications, the potential for drug interactions and the paucity of controlled studies examining the efficacy of current asthma treatments in older adults.

Background

Although asthma is commonly thought of as a disease of children and young adults, a significant percentage (4-13%) of the older adult (>65 years old) population in the United States is affected [1]. The prevalence of asthma in older adults may even be higher as studies have shown that asthma is often underdiagnosed in this growing population. Older adults with asthma also carry a greater burden of morbidity and mortality of the disease with one study noting a 3-fold increase in the death rate among the oldest adults in comparison to younger adults [2, 3]. In addition to this increased morbidity and mortality, asthma in older adults can be challenging to diagnose due to multiple comorbid conditions and the broad differential diagnosis of other diseases that can produce symptoms similar to asthma. Furthermore, there is inadequate use of pulmonary function tests in older adults, which often leads to a delay in the diagnosis [4]. This review will focus on the pathogenesis, complications, and management of asthma in older adults.

Impact of Asthma in Older Adults

The morbidity and mortality of asthma in older adults is significant, with more than 2000 asthma related deaths in older adults each year in the United States [5]. The prevalence of asthma and mortality due to asthma in all age groups has been steadily increasing since 1980, with a peak in mortality in 1998. In comparison to older males, females have an increased prevalence of asthma and higher mortality rates [5, 6]. Adults older than 65 years are more likely to use medical resources and treatment for asthma. Furthermore, they are noted to have increased hospitalizations, emergency department visits and outpatient visits [7-10].

Asthma has a significant impact on the quality of life of those affected by it. Inadequate treatment in older adults is common, despite its known impact on quality of life. In the Cardiovascular Health Study, 35% of older adults with asthma were reported to have a fair or poor health status compared to 17% of non-asthmatic older adults [11-14]. Despite a diagnosis of definite asthma, only 40% of older adults were treated with a rescue albuterol inhaler, and only 30% were treated with an inhaled corticosteroid [11-14].

Pathogenesis

Asthma is defined as a chronic inflammatory disease associated with variable airflow obstruction and bronchial hyperresponsiveness, both of which are reversible in most patients. Airway inflammation is a central feature of asthma and is mediated by numerous inflammatory cells (eosinophils, neutrophils, T_H2 lymphocytes, basophils, and mast cells) that infiltrate the airways [15]. These inflammatory cells may be activated by a particular insult (e.g. upper respiratory infection or allergen exposure) and results in a release of mediators, including cytokines, chemokines, and lipid mediators. The release of inflammatory mediators increases cellular activation and recruitment of additional inflammatory cells, promotes mucus secretion, and induces bronchoconstriction. This series of events produces the symptoms of asthma, including cough, shortness of breath and wheezing.

Despite general familiarity with the molecular mechanisms of asthma, the pathogenesis of asthma in older adults is not well understood. Asthma in older adults may result from the persistence of childhood asthma (long-standing asthma: LSA), recurrence of childhood asthma formerly in remission, or the development of asthma later in life (late-onset asthma: LOA). LSA is characterized by the onset of symptoms early in life, a higher incidence of atopy, more severe obstruction with less bronchodilator reversibility and greater hyperinflation [16,17]. In contrast, the symptoms of LOA occur in middle age or older. Patients with LOA have a decreased incidence of atopy, a greater response to bronchodilators and a higher baseline FEV_1 [16,17]. Thus, the duration of asthma appears to have a role in the severity and the development of irreversible airflow obstruction [16]. Many questions regarding the different mechanisms of these two phenotypes of asthma in older adults remain unanswered, and shedding light on these research questions will impact current practices in the diagnosis and treatment of asthma in older adults. Table 1 highlights the differences between long standing asthma and late onset asthma.

The role of allergen sensitization, genetics and environmental exposures are not clearly defined in LOA and persistence of asthma in older adults.

Studies examining the natural history of asthma in older adults reveal lower total IgE levels, fewer positive skin prick test responses and less concomitant atopic diseases [18]. Despite this, the relationship between IgE levels and allergic disease persists in older adults with some reports indicating up to 72% of newly diagnosed older asthmatics had evidence of elevated total IgE and/or antigen-specific IgE [19,20]. Moreover, sensitization to certain allergens, such as cockroach allergens, is associated with more severe asthma in older adults [21]. Although family history is an important risk factor for childhood asthma, its significance in LOA is not as clear. Mitsunobu and colleagues examined the role of family history in bronchial hyper-responsiveness in older individuals (age 50-59 years old) and found that those with a family history of asthma had greater bronchial hyper-responsiveness [22]. In young children and infants, viral infections such as RSV are known to be causes of asthma exacerbations and wheezing. The common upper respiratory viral pathogens precipitating acute cardiopulmonary hospitalizations in adults include influenza A, RSV, and human metapneumovirus (hMPV). However, many of these patients have underlying heart and lung conditions. Frequent episodes of viral infections triggering asthma exacerbations may lead to LOA, but whether this is mediated by the infections themselves or underlying susceptibilities, such as lung disease, remains to be determined.

Table 1. Long Standing Asthma (LSA) vs. Late Onset Asthma (LOA) [Adapted from reference: 14]

	LSA	**LOA**
Age of Onset	Age< 40 years	Age> 40 years
Infections	Viral	Viral and Bacterial
Allergy	Likely	Unlikely
Inflammation	T_H2 driven Eosinophilic	T_H1 or T_H2 driven Neutrophilic and/or Eosinophilic
Environment	Allergens, daycare, school, and workplace	Workplace, dwelling type (house, apartment, institutional)

Irrespective of the presence of lung disease, normal aging is associated with changes in lung function that potentiate the effects of asthma (Table 2). The prevalence of airway hyperresponsiveness increases with age and is linked with a reduction in lung function, a history of smoking, and inflammatory mechanisms [23]. With each year of life after age 20, there is a continuous 25 to 30 ml decrease in FEV_1 and FVC. The variability in pulmonary physiology due to aging in conjunction with asthma has been shown to lead to a greater decline in lung function in aging asthmatics in comparison to healthy individuals [24]. The basis for this decrease in lung function in asthma is airway hyperresponsiveness, which results in an increase in residual volume (RV) leading to a decrease in FVC and FEV_1. There are several potential factors that account for the increase in airway reactivity seen with aging. First, age has been associated with an increase in the neuronal mechanisms, which control bronchial smooth muscle contractility [23]. Long-term exposure to tobacco smoking or environmental factors can release immune mediators from respiratory epithelium that can cause an increase in bronchial smooth muscle contractility. Additionally, imbalances between non-adrenergic inhibitory and non-cholinergic excitatory fibers have been cited as possible causes of increased bronchial tone. Finally, the age-related decrease in β-adrenergic receptor function also contributes to the increased airway reactivity seen in older asthmatics.

In addition to affecting pulmonary function, aging influences the structure and physiology of the lungs themselves, which may exacerbate the effects of asthma. As a consequence of aging, there is a compromise in lung structure with homogenous airspace enlargement and decreased elastic lung recoil pressure [23]. The decreased lung elastic recoil results in enhanced airway bronchoconstriction and the loss of radial traction in the airway walls leads to a reduction in maximal expiratory flow rates (FEV_1) that can lead to an increase in RV [23].

Another pathophysiological consequence of aging is a decreased perception of bronchoconstriction, which may contribute to the increase in asthma related morbidity. This decrease in perception of bronchoconstriction has been demonstrated in studies of both healthy and asthmatic older adults. In both studies, subjects underwent methacholine bronchoprovocation study and despite similar falls in FVC to younger adults, the older adults were less likely to perceive the significant decline in lung function [25, 26]. Moreover, in the older asthmatics larger falls in FVC occurred, which suggests an increase in lung inflation and bronchoconstriction [25]. Comorbid conditions in older adults further confound the ability of older asthmatics to perceive bronchoconstriction, which has been shown to limit the quality of life [25]. Neuronal mechanisms also contribute the decreased awareness of bronchoconstriction seen in older adults. Older adults have deterioration in the sensitivity and accuracy of inspiratory proprioception which results in a diminished ventilatory response to hypoxia and hypercapnia, making older asthmatics more vulnerable to respiratory failure during high demand states [24].

Lastly, immune cell function has been shown to decrease with age, a property often termed "immunosenescence", which may have implications in asthma [27]. The inflammatory cells affected include neutrophils, dendritic cells, eosinophils, macrophages, T cells and B cells. Changes in the function of these key immune players may alter an individual's ability to clear pathogens as well as impact baseline airway inflammation. Given that inflammation is the cornerstone of asthma, it is of interest to determine how the airway inflammation in older asthmatics differs from those of their younger counterparts. These changes may impact the susceptibility to exacerbations by pathogens and the treatment response at baseline and during an exacerbation.

Table 2. Special Features of Asthma in Older Adults

1. **Increased Airway Reactivity** • Increased neuronal mechanism • Long term tobacco and environmental exposure • Imbalance between non adrenergic inhibitory and non cholinergic excitatory fibers • Decreased beta adrenergic receptor function
2. **Lung Structure and Function** • Decreased lung compliance • Decreased elastic recoil • Decreased respiratory muscle strength
3. **Decreased Sensation of Bronchoconstriction** • Comorbid conditions are confounding factors • Decreased sensitivity of inspiratory proprioception • Diminished ventilatory response to hypoxia and hypercapnia
4. **Immunosenescence** • Decreased immune cell function • Increased airway neutrophilia and increased $CD4^+$ T cells • Decreased eosinophil effector function of degranulation and superoxide production • Decreased sputum expression of leukotriene B_4

Diagnosis of Asthma in Older Adults

At first glance, older asthmatics share several characteristics with their younger counterparts. The presenting symptoms of asthma in older adults are similar to those in younger age groups and include episodic wheezing, shortness of breath, and chest tightness. These symptoms are more prominent at nighttime or during exertional activities. Asthma symptoms are often triggered by upper respiratory infections, environmental exposures (i.e. environmental tobacco smoke, aeroallergens, and strong odors) and medications (i.e. aspirin, non-steroidal anti-inflammatory agents, β-blockers, or angiotensin-converting enzyme inhibitors). As the older adult population commonly uses many of these medications it is imperative to review medications that older asthmatics are taking.

However, despite these similarities in clinical presentation, certain complexities emerge when dealing with asthma in older adults compared to their younger counterparts. The older adult population has a significant number of comorbid conditions, which have symptoms that may overlap or even mimic asthma symptoms. Many different diagnoses must be considered when evaluating an older adult for asthma. These include congestive heart failure, COPD, chronic aspiration, gastroesophageal reflux disease and pulmonary embolism (Table 3). Thus it is imperative to also use objective measures when diagnosing asthma in older adults.

One such measure is pulmonary function testing (PFT), which is a powerful tool in diagnosis of asthma in older adults [28,29]. One misconception about PFTs, which results in underutilization in this population, is that older adults are not able to perform PFTs adequately. However, studies report that 80% to 90% of patients aged $>$ 65 years can perform PFTs successfully when tested by a skilled technologist [29-34]. However, there are some important caveats about the use of pulmonary function testing in older adults. First, older adults with cognitive or physical impairments may not be able to perform spirometry effectively. Second, predicted normal values of spirometry parameters are often different in older individuals. For example, using a FEV1/FVC ratio < 0.70 (based on Global initiative for Obstructive Lung Disease guidelines) to define obstructive lung disease can lead to a high rate of misclassification in the elderly, since the predicted normal values and ratio may be lower in this population [14,34]. The correct approach is to use the lower limit of the normal range of FEV1/FVC, based on the fifth percentile corrected for age, sex, height, and race. In order to account for lung compromise in older adults, the lower limit of a normal FEV1/FVC should be <0.60 in 85-yr-old people, and not 0.70 [36,37]. Using FEV_6 (forced expiratory volume in six seconds) as an alternative to FVC has also been suggested, since it provides a better estimate of forced vital capacity and reduces misinterpretation [37].

PFTs may not always be the best tool to assess airway hyperresponsiveness as it may not be present during testing. Methacholine challenge can be used to assess airway hyperresponsiveness. However, in older asthmatics that may have developed fixed airflow obstruction, methacholine challenge may not be a useful diagnostic tool [38-41]. Additionally, some studies have shown that bronchial responsiveness is heightened in older adults and thus age may independently influence airway responsiveness [23,14].

Table 3. Differential diagnosis of asthma in older adults

Pulmonary	Cardiovascular	Neoplastic	Other
Chronic obstructive pulmonary disease	Pulmonary embolism	Lung Cancer	Aspiration
Asthma	Atrial fibrillation	Endobronchial Tumors	Gastro-esophageal reflux
Bronchiectasis	Coronary heart disease	Endotracheal Tumors	Vocal cord dysfunction
Pulmonary vascular disease	Cardiovascular deconditioning	Lymphoma with hilar adenopathy	Mechanical airway obstruction
Restrictive lung disease	Heart failure		Obesity
Upper airway obstruction			
Constrictive bronchiolitis			
Chronic Cough			
Churg-Strauss Syndrome			

A concomitant diagnosis of asthma and COPD is common among older adults. One study has reported up to 50% of older adults with obstructive lung disease have features of both asthma and COPD [42]. According to National Health and Nutrition Examination Survey (NHANES) III, participants with a diagnosis of both asthma and COPD have a higher prevalence of objective airflow obstruction, in comparison to patients with a diagnosis of emphysema-alone [43,44].

Unlike most cases of COPD, however, the airflow obstruction in asthma is typically reversible, though there is a tendency for this to diminish with age. In fact, approximately 30% of patients with fixed airflow obstruction have a history of asthma [44]. Reversibility of airflow obstruction in asthma is defined as post-bronchodilator FEV_1 or FVC increases of >12% and 200 mL after inhalation of a short-acting β-agonist, such as albuterol. This reversibility is often blunted in older asthmatics due to a reduced number of β-adrenergic receptors on smooth airway muscles. To complicate matters, some studies have shown that bronchial responsiveness is heightened in older adults [14]. Together, these factors contribute to the difficulty in differentiating asthma from COPD in older individuals using conventional diagnostic methods.

The gross changes in lung structure and function in asthma begin at the cellular level. Asthmatics regardless of having variable or fixed airflow obstruction have a unique profile of cellular infiltrates and an increased thickness of reticular layer of basement membrane compared to patients with COPD **(Figure 1)** [43]. In asthmatics, $CD4^+$ T_H2 lymphocytes have a prominent role in mediating the inflammatory cascade. Airway infiltration is marked with eosinophils and $CD4^+$ lymphocytes causing airway remodeling, microvascular leaks, excessive formation of mucus and exudates, epithelial disruption and increased numbers of epithelial goblet cells. This leads to airflow obstruction and interstitial collagen deposition beneath the epithelium. In contrast, $CD8^+$ T_H1 lymphocytes have a more important role in mediating the inflammatory cascade in patients with COPD. Airway infiltration is characterized by neutrophils and $CD8^+$ lymphocytes causing airway remodeling accompanied by goblet cell metaplasia, mucous plugging, smooth muscle hypertrophy and airway wall fibrosis and distortion that narrow and obliterate the airway lumen. [24,43]

Non-invasive diagnostic tests such as sputum induction (presence of sputum eosinophils >3%) and exhaled nitric oxide (>16 ppb) may be clinically useful in distinguishing asthma from COPD in elderly patients without clear clinical history or in those with multiple risk factors [43]. Moreover, asthmatics are observed to have a higher diffusing capacity and PaO_2, and a lower residual volume and high-resolution CT (HRCT) emphysema score. This is consistent with less lung parenchymal involvement in asthma. In comparison, COPD patients tend to have a low diffusing capacity and PaO_2, higher residual volume and higher HRCT emphysema score; consistent with increased lung parenchymal destruction [43].

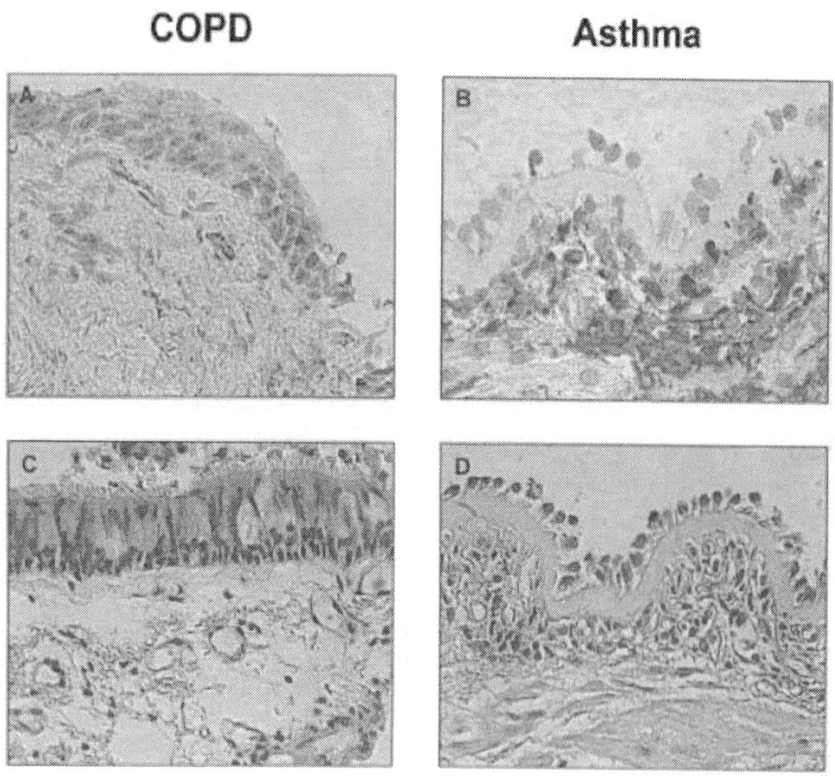

Figure 1. Pathology of fixed airflow obstruction in COPD (A) and asthma (B), immunostained with anti-EG2 (eosinophil cationic protein). H&E stain depicting fixed airflow obstruction in patients with COPD (C) and asthma (D). A thicker reticular layer of epithelial basement membrane is noted in asthma (D) compared with COPD (C). Reprinted with permission of the American Thoracic Society. Copyright © 2011 American Thoracic Society. Cite: Fabbri LM, Romagnoli M, Corbetta L, Casoni G, Busljetic K, Turato G, Ligabue G, Ciaccia A, Saetta M, Papi A. Differences in Airway Inflammation in Patients with Fixed Airflow Obstruction Due to Asthma or Chronic Obstructive Pulmonary Disease. *Am J Respir Crit Care Med* 2003; 167: 418-424.

Management of Asthma in Older Adults

The management of asthma in all age groups focuses on the assessment and monitoring of asthma control, asthma education for a partnership in care, control of environmental factors, control of co-morbid factors and pharmacologic therapy [45]. The 2007 NHLBI guidelines however, recognize that older adults have special needs particularly in asthma education and medication use. Asthma management in older adults can be challenging as they are at increased risk for adverse reactions than younger patients [30]. These special considerations will be reviewed in this section.

The goal of asthma therapy is to achieve well-controlled asthma by reducing the frequency and severity of both symptoms and exacerbations, maintaining normal levels of activity and achieving optimal lung function. Asthma severity is determined prior to the initiation of treatment and is based on symptom frequency and objective measures of lung function. Severity can be classified as intermittent or persistent. Intermittent asthma is defined as no interference with daily activities, daytime symptoms occurring <2 times per week and/or nighttime symptoms occurring <2 times per month. In persistent asthma, there is a limitation of daily activities, more frequent symptoms and use of rescue medications. Moreover, persistent asthma is classified into mild, moderate and severe, based on a patient's level of impairment. Asthma control is assessed once therapy has been initiated and is subsequently monitored every 1-6 months to determine if the goals of therapy have been met and if adjustment to therapy (i.e., step up or step down) is necessary [45]. Control is assessed using both subjective (i.e. administration of standardized questionnaires or asking questions about sleep impairments and difficulty with daily activities due to asthma) and objective (i.e. spirometry or peak flow) measures. The subjective measures may be difficult to evaluate in older patients as they have a poorer perception of their asthma symptoms when compared to their younger counterparts and they often attribute symptoms such as dyspnea to aging [46].

Home peak expiratory flow (PEF) monitoring is commonly used to evaluate asthma control and may be helpful in patients with co-morbidities such as heart or lung disease, as these diseases can mimic symptoms of asthma. However, the benefit of home monitoring in the older adult population may be limited as age-related changes in lung mechanics, airway structure and a decline in physical and cognitive function that affect the patient's ability to perform the PEF maneuver. Studies reflect that PEF measurement may be beneficial if the older adult is highly motivated and is able to attain twice daily measurements for few weeks [47-49].

Asthma education is a necessary component of asthma management. Complex medication regimens, memory loss and cognitive dysfunction all contribute to poor compliance and adherence to treatment in older asthmatics making asthma education critical. [30,50,51]. Increasing age has been shown to be a factor in determining the correct use of inhaler devices (Table 4). Incorrect use is often secondary to decreased muscle strength, memory problems and a loss of coordination [51]. Meter dose inhalers (MDIs) can be difficult for older adults to use due to arthritis or the proper synchronization of hand actuation and inspiration needed for effective drug delivery [51]. Patients with arthritis may do better with breath-activated delivery devices instead. However, a significant number of older adults are unable to generate adequate peak inspiratory flow for the optimal use of some popular dry powder inhaler (DPI) devices [14]. The relationship between poor inspiratory flow and age is multifactorial and ranges from the severity of asthma to proper nutrition and co-existing conditions. Once these barriers to medication delivery are recognized, the health care provider and/or asthma educator can tailor education on device handling to each individual. This can improve adherence to treatment and may allow individuals to maintain and live an independent, active and personally satisfying life.

The identification of environmental triggers and co-morbid conditions can aid in attaining asthma control in both young and older asthmatics. Common environmental triggers include aeroallergens, respiratory infections and irritants (i.e. tobacco smoke, pollution, chemicals, and cold air). Aeroallergen sensitization can by examined by allergy skin testing or specific IgE measurement in the blood. Sensitization to indoor allergens may have a greater impact in older adults, as they tend to spend more time indoors [52]. Thus, it is essential to discuss measures to reduce allergen exposure with patients that exhibit allergen sensitivity.

Several other diseases, which are prevalent in the older adult population, can have a significant impact on asthma control. Gastroesophageal reflux disease (GERD) can exacerbate asthma symptoms and in one report it was present in up to 80% of asthmatics [53]. Obesity has also been associated with an increased prevalence and severity of asthma [54]. Furthermore, a reduction in weight has been shown to improve asthma symptoms [55].

Table 4. Strategies for Overcoming Barriers to Compliance with Medications in Older Adults [Adapted from: reference 30]

Barriers to Compliance	Therapeutic Strategies
Arthritis of Hands and Fingers	• Avoid metered dose inhalers (MDI) • Use breath activated delivery systems
Depression	• Identify and treat affective disorder
Poor Memory	• Keep regimens as simple as possible • Use written action plans in large print
Limited or Fixed Income	• Bear drug costs in mind when prescribing
Visual Impairment	• Use color coding • Use enlarged fonts for medication instructions

The recommendations for the treatment of asthma in older adults are not much different than for younger adults. The most recent NHLBI asthma guidelines acknowledge that anticholinergic medications may have a greater role in older adults [45]. Additionally, the guidelines point out that health care providers should recognize potential side effects and drug interactions that could impact asthma such as β-blockers (Table 5). β-blockers are commonly used in older adults and can provoke bronchospasm, though the use of cardioselective β-blockers has a much lower incidence of bronchospasm than the non-selective β-blockers (i.e. propranolol, nadolol and esmolol) [56]. Ophthalmologic solutions containing non-selective β-blockers (i.e. timolol) should be avoided as they may produce a fatal asthma attack [57]. Aspirin and NSAIDs may also lead to acute bronchospasm in those with aspirin sensitive asthma. Angiotensin converting enzyme inhibitors may lead to dry cough further worsening symptoms of asthma.

Bronchodilators are first line treatment for acute symptomatic control of asthma. Stimulation of β-2 adrenergic receptors leads to an increase in sympathetic system activity, reduction in adenylyl cyclase responses and increased inhibitory G protein expression. This cascade of events leads to smooth muscle relaxation and bronchial dilatation. Side effects of short-acting β-agonists (SABAs) include tachycardia, tremor, a dose dependent decrease in serum potassium levels and dose dependent prolongation of the QT interval on EKG [58]. Due to different age related physiologic response to β-adrenergic receptor stimulation, these side effects are more pronounced in older adults [14, 58, 59].

Table 5. Medication Considerations in Older Adults

Pharmacotherapy	Side Effect in Older Adults	Alternative Therapy
Non-cardioselective β-blocker	• Bronchospasm	Selective β blocker
Topical β-blocker (ophthalmic solution)	• Fatal asthma attack	
Bronchodilator: short-acting β-agonists	• Tachycardia, tremor, a dose dependent decrease in serum potassium levels • Dose dependent prolongation of the QT interval on EKG	
Aspirin and NSAIDs	• Avoid use in patients with Aspirin sensitivity	Acetaminophen
Angiotensin Converting Enzyme Inhibitor (ACEI)	• Increased dry cough	Angiotensin Receptor Blocker (ARB)
Anticholinergics	• Increased dry mouth, urinary hesitancy, constipation and increased ocular pressure. • Avoid use in patients with glaucoma	Use a spacer with MDI and a mouthpiece (when used with nebulized form)
Theophylline	• Increased toxicity: seizures, atrial fibrillation, supraventricular tachycardia, ventricular ectopy and ventricular tachycardia	
Systemic corticosteroids	• Increased risk of bone fractures, cataracts, muscle weakness, back pain, bruising and oral candidiasis. • Provokes confusion, agitation and glucose metabolism changes	Inhaled corticosteroid
Inhaled corticosteroids	• Local adverse effects: hoarseness, dysphonia, cough, oral candidiasis	Use a spacer

Anticholinergics may be an effective alternative to long-acting β-agonists (LABAs) in the older adult population. The adverse effects of anticholinergic medications, such as dry mouth, urinary hesitancy, constipation, and increased ocular pressure are especially notable in older adults. Additionally, caution should be used in patients with glaucoma. To limit deposition in the eye, a spacer should be used with the MDI and a mouthpiece, not a facemask, should be used when administering the nebulized form [57,60].

Theophylline should be used cautiously in older adults due to its narrow therapeutic range and toxic events. Aging is associated with decreased activity of the enzyme phosphodiestrase as well as changes in liver and kidney function causes reduced clearance and increased half-life of the drug. Theophylline toxicity can lead to seizures, atrial fibrillation, supraventricular tachycardia, ventricular ectopy and ventricular tachycardia.

Oral glucocorticoids may be used as a diagnostic tool to assess difference between reversible or fixed airway obstructions in older individuals, when bronchodilator therapy may not be effective [45]. However, the use of systemic corticosteroids can have deleterious effects in the older adult population with an increased risk of bone fractures, cataracts, muscle weakness, back pain, bruising, and oral candidiasis [61]. Additionally, they can provoke confusion, agitation, and changes in glucose metabolism. Inhaled corticosteroids may be a better alternative for use in older adults but it may cause local adverse effects such as hoarseness, dysphonia, cough and oral candidiasis, which can be reduced with the use of a spacer.

Conclusion

Though asthma is most common in children or young adults (8-10%), the prevalence of asthma in older adults (>65 years old) is increasing and expected to double in the next 20 years [2,3]. Despite this increase in prevalence, it is underdiagnosed and undertreated. The diagnosis of asthma in older adults can be challenging due to a decrease in the perception of symptoms and coexisting conditions such as congestive heart failure and chronic obstructive pulmonary disease. Despite evidence that the airway inflammation in older adults with asthma differs from that of younger adults, the management of the disease is very similar. When treating older asthmatics, special attention should be made to the adverse effects of asthma medications as well as potentially serious drug interactions. There are obvious gaps in our current knowledge of asthma in older adults and further research is needed to allow us to provide personalized care to the growing aging population.

References

[1] Busse PJ; Kilaru K. *Complexities of Diagnosis and Treatment of Allergic Respiratory Disease in the Elderly.* Drugs & Aging, 2009. 26(1): p. 1-22

[2] Robin ED. Death from bronchial asthma. *Chest* 1988; 93 (3): 614-8

[3] Slavin, R.G.; et al. Asthma in older adults: observations from the Epidemiology and Natural History of Asthma: Outcomes and treatment regimens (TENOR) study. *Annals of Allergy Asthma & Immunology,* 2006. 96(3): 406-414

[4] Bauer BA; Reed CE; Yunginger JW; Wollan PC; Silverstein MD. Incidence and outcomes of asthma in the elderly. A population-based study in Rochester, Minnesota. *Chest* 1997;111: 303-10.

[5] CDC. National surveillance for asthma---United States, 1980--2004. In: *Surveillance Summaries,* October 19, 2007. MMWR 2007; 56(No. SS-8).

[6] Moorman JE; Mannino DM. Increasing U.S. asthma mortality rates: who is really dying? *J Asthma* 2001; 38:65.

[7] Barr RG; Somers SC; Speizer FE; Camargo CA Jr. Patient factors and medication guideline adherence among older women with asthma. *Arch Intern Med* 2002; 162:1761-8.

[8] Krigsman K; Moen J; Nilsson JL; Ring L. Refill adherence by the elderly for asthma/chronic obstructive pulmonary disease drugs dispensed over a 10-year period. *J Clin Pharm Ther* 2007;32: 603-11.

[9] Kung HC; Hoyert DL; Xu J; Murphy SL. Deaths: final data for 2005. *Natl Vital Stat Rep* 2008;56: 1-120.

[10] Zeiger RS; Hay JW; Contreras R; Chen W; Quinn VP; Seal B; et al. Asthma costs and utilization in a managed care organization. *J Allergy Clin Immunol* 2008;121: 885-92.

[11] Enright PL; McClelland RL; Newman AB; et al. Underdiagnosis and undertreatment of asthma in the elderly. Cardiovascular Health Study Research Group. *Chest* 1999; 116:603.

[12] Enright PL; Ward BJ; Tracy RP; Lasser EC. Asthma and its association with cardiovascular disease in the elderly. The Cardiovascular Health Study Research Group. *J Asthma* 1996;33: 45-53.

[13] Fried LP; Borhani NO; Enright P; Furberg CD; Gardin JM; Kronmal RA; et al. The Cardiovascular Health Study: design and rationale. *Ann Epidemiol* 1991;1: 263-76.

[14] Hanania NA; King MJ; Braman SS; Saltoun C; Wise RA; Enright P; Falsey AR; Mathur SK; Ramsdell JW; Rogers L; Stempel DA; Lima JJ; Fish JE; Wilson SR; Boyd C; Patel KV; Irvin CG; Yawn BP; Halm EA; Wasserman SI; Sands MF; Ershler WB; Ledford DK. Asthma in the elderly: Current understanding and future research needs--a report of a National Institute on Aging (NIA) workshop. *J Allergy Clin Immunol.* 2011 Sep;128(3 Suppl): S4-24.

[15] Drazen, JM; Arm, JP; Austen, KF. Sorting out the cytokines of asthma. *J Exp Med,* 1996. 183(1): 1-5.

[16] Cassino C; Berger KI; Goldring RM; Norman RG; Kammerman S; Ciotoli C; Reibman J. Duration of asthma and physiologic outcomes in elderly nonsmokers. *Am J Respir Crit Care Med.* 2000 Oct;162(4 Pt 1):1423-8.

[17] Braman SS; Kamerlen JT; Davis SM. Asthma in Elderly: A comparison between patients with recently acquired and long-standing disease. *Am Rev Respir Dis 1992*;143: 336.

[18] Slavin, R.G.; et al.. Asthma in older adults: observations from the Epidemiology and Natural History of Asthma: Outcomes and treatment regimens (TENOR) study. *Annals of Allergy Asthma & Immunology,* 2006. 96(3): 406-414.

[19] Busse, P.J.. Allergic Respiratory Disease in the Elderly. *The American Journal of Medicine,* 2007. 120(6): 498-502.

[20] Litonjua, AA; et al.. Sensitization to Cat Allergen Is Associated with Asthma in Older Men and Predicts New-onset Airway Hyperresponsiveness . The Normative Aging Study. *Am. J. Respir. Crit. Care Med.,* 1997. 156(1): 23-27.

[21] Rogers L; Cassino C; Berger KI; et al. Asthma in the elderly: cockroach sensitization and severity of airway obstruction in elderly nonsmokers. *Chest* 2002; 122 (5): 1580-6.

[22] Mitsunobu F; Mifune T; Hosaki Y; Ashida K; Tsugeno H; Okamoto M; Harada S; Tanizaki Y. IgE-mediated and age-related bronchial hyperresponsiveness in patients with asthma relationship to family history of the disease. *Age Ageing.* 2000 May;29(3):215-20.

[23] Scichilone N; M. Messina; S. Nattaglia; F. Catalano; V. Bellia. Airway hyperresponsiveness in the elderly: prevalence and clinical implications. *Eur Respir J* 2005: 364-75.

[24] Sharma G; Goodwin J. Effect of aging on respiratory system physiology and immunology. *Clin Interv Aging.* 2006;1(3): 253-60.

[25] Cuttitta G; Cibella F; Bellia V; et al. Changes in FVC during methacholine-induced bronchoconstriction in elderly patients with asthma: bronchial hyper responsiveness and aging. *Chest.* 2001;119: 1685–90.

[26] Connolly MJ; Crowley JJ; Charan NB; Nielson CP; Vestal RE. Reduced subjective awareness of bronchoconstriction provoked by methacholine in elderly asthmatic and normal subjects as measured on a simple awareness scale. *Thorax* 1992;47: 410-3.

[27] Aw, D.; A.B. Silva; D.B. Palmer. Immunosenescence: emerging challenges for an ageing population. *Immunology,* 2007. 120(4): 435-446

[28] Enright PL; Kronmal RA; Higgins M; et al. Spirometry reference values for women and men 65 to 85 years of age. Cardiovascular health study. *Am Rev Respir Dis* 1993; 147:125.

[29] Enright PL; Burchette RJ; Peters JA; Lebowitz MD; McDonnell WF; Abbey DE. Peak flow lability: association with asthma and spirometry in an older cohort. *Ches*t 1997;112: 895-901.

[30] Braman SS; Hanania NA. Asthma in older adults. *Clin Chest Med.* 2007 Dec; 28: 685-702.

[31] Quadrelli SA; Roncoroni A. Features of asthma in the elderly. *J Asthma* 2001; 38:377.

[32] Lehmann S; Vollset SE; Nygaard HA; Gulsvik A. Factors determining performance of bronchodilator reversibility tests in middle-aged and elderly. *Respir Med* 2004;98: 1071-9.

[33] Pezzoli L; Giardini G; Consonni S; Dallera I; Bilotta C; Ferrario G; et al. Quality of spirometric performance in older people. *Age Ageing* 2003;32: 43-6.

[34] De Fillipi F; Tana F; Vanzati S; Balzarini B; Galetti G. Study of respiratory function in the elderly with different nutritional and cognitive status and functional ability assessed by plethysmographic and spirometric parameters. *Arch Gerontol Geriatr* 2003;37: 33-43.

[35] Bellia V; Pistelli R; Catalano F; Antonelli-Incalzi R; Grassi V; Melillo G; et al. Quality control of spirometry in the elderly. The SA.R.A. study. Salute Respiration nell'Anziano 5 Respiratory Health in the Elderly. *Am J Respir Crit Care Med* 2000;161: 1094-100.

[36] Hansen EF; Phanareth K; Laursen LC; Kok-Jensen A; Dirksen A. Reversible and irreversible airflow obstruction as predictor of overall

mortality in asthma and chronic obstructive pulmonary disease. *Am J Respir Crit Care Med* 1999;159: 1267-71.

[37] Hankinson JL; Odencrantz JR; Fedan KB. Spirometric reference values from a sample of the general U.S. population. *Am J Respir Crit Care Med* 1999; 159:179.

[38] Hargreave FE; O'Byrne PM; Ramsdale EH. Mediators, airway responsiveness, and asthma. *J Allergy Clin Immunol* 1985;76: 272–276.

[39] Tashkin DP; Altose MD; Bleecker ER; Connett JE; Kanner RE; Lee WW; Wise R. The lung health study: airway responsiveness to inhaled methacholine in smokers with mild to moderate airflow limitation: The Lung Health Study Research Group. *Am Rev Respir Dis* 1992;145: 301–310.

[40] Kanner RE; Connett JE; Altose MD; Buist AS; Lee WW; Tashkin DP; Wise RA.Gender difference in airway hyperresponsiveness in smokers with mild COPD: The Lung Health Study. *Am J Respir Crit Care Med* 1994;150: 956–961.

[41] Crapo RO; Casaburi R; Coates AL; Enright PL; Hankinson JL; Irvin CG; MacIntyre NR; McKay RT; Wanger JS; Anderson SD; et al. Guidelines for methacholine and exercise challenge testing:1999. *Am. J Respir Crit Care Med* 2000;161: 309–329.

[42] Soriano JB; Davis KJ; Coleman B; Visick G; Mannino D; Pride NB. The proportional Venn diagram of obstructive lung disease: two approximations from the United States and the United Kingdom. *CHEST* 2003;124: 474-81.

[43] Fabbri LM; Romagnoli M; Corbetta L; Casoni G; Busljetic K; Turato G; Ligabue G; Ciaccia A; Saetta M; Papi A. Differences in Airway Inflammation in Patients with Fixed Airflow Obstruction Due to Asthma or Chronic Obstructive Pulmonary Disease. *Am J Respir Crit Care Med* 2003; 167: 418-424.

[44] Mannino DM; Gagnon RC; Petty TL; Lydick E. Obstructive lung disease and low lung function in adults in the United States: data from the National Health and Nutrition Examination Survey, 1988-1994. *Arch Intern Med* 2000; 160: 1683-1689.

[45] National Asthma Education and Prevention Program: Expert panel report III: *Guidelines for the diagnosis and management of asthma.* Bethesda, MD: National Heart, Lung, and Blood Institute, 2007. (NIH publication no. 08-4051)

[46] Ekici A; Ekici M; Bulcun E. Affect status and perception of exacerbation in patients with asthma. *Allergy Asthma Proc.* 2010 Nov-Dec;31(6):106-10.

[47] Enright PL. The diagnosis and management of asthma is much tougher in older patients. *Curr Opin Allergy Clin Immunol* 2002; 2:175.

[48] Künzli N; Stutz EZ; Perruchoud AP; et al. Peak flow variability in the SAPALDIA study and its validity in screening for asthma-related conditions. The SPALDIA Team. *Am J Respir Crit Care Med* 1999; 160:427.

[49] Goldstein MF; Veza BA; Dunsky EH; et al. Comparisons of peak diurnal expiratory flow variation, postbronchodilator FEV(1) responses, and methacholine inhalation challenges in the evaluation of suspected asthma. *Chest* 2001; 119:1001.

[50] King MJ; Hanania NA. Asthma in the elderly: current knowledge and future directions. *Curr Opin Pulm Med* 2010;16: 55-9.

[51] Molimard M; Raherison C; Lignot S; Depont F; Abouelfath A; Moore N. Assessment of handling of inhaler devices in real life: an observational study in 3811 patients in primary care. *J Aerosol Med.* 2003 Fall;16(3): 249-54.

[52] Rogers L; Cassino C; Berger KI; et al. Asthma in the elderly: cockroach sensitization and severity of airway obstruction in elderly nonsmokers. *Chest* 2002; 122 (5): 1580-6.

[53] Harding SM; Guzzo MR; Richter JE. The prevalence of gastroesophageal reflux in asthma patients without reflux symptoms. *Am J Respir Crit Care Med* 2000; 162 (1): 34-9.

[54] Weiss ST. Obesity: insight into the origins of asthma. *Nat Immunol* 2005; 6 (6): 537-9.

[55] Stenius-Aarniala B; Poussa T; Kvarnstrom J; et al. Immediate and long term effects of weight reduction in obese people with asthma: randomised controlled study. *BMJ* 2000; 320 (7238): 827-32.

[56] Salpeter S; Ormiston T; Salpeter E. Cardioselective beta-blocker use in patients with reactive airway disease: a meta-analysis. *Ann Intern Med.* 2002;137: 715-725.

[57] Odeh M; Oliven A; Bassan H. Timolol eye drop-induced fatal bronchospasm in an asthmatic patient. *J Fam Pract* 1991; 32 (1): 97-8.

[58] Gupta P; O'Mahony S . Potential Adverse Effects of Bronchodilators in the Treatment of Airways Obstruction in Older People: Recommendations for Prescribing. *Drugs Aging* 2008; 25(29): 415–443.

[59] Connolly MJ; Crowley JJ; Charan NB; Nielson CP; Vestal RE. Impaired bronchodilator response to albuterol in healthy elderly men and women. *Chest.* 1995 Aug;108(2):401-6.

[60] Newnham DM. Asthma medications and their potential adverse effects in the elderly: recommendations for prescribing. *Drug Saf* 2001; 24 (14): 1065-80.

[61] Walsh LJ; Wong CA; Oborne J; Cooper S; Lewis SA; Pringle M; et al. Adverse Effects of Oral corticosteroids in relation to dose inpatients with lung function. *Thorax* 2001; 56: 279.

In: Asthma: Causes, Complications and Treatment ISBN: 978-1-62257-447-6
Editors: A. H. Bislimi and L. C. Tolka

Chapter IV

Changes of Respiratory Epithelium in Bronchial Asthma

Adriana Grigoraş and Irina-Draga Căruntu
Department of Histology, "Gr. T. Popa" University of Medicine and Pharmacy, Iaşi, Romania

Abstract

Airway epithelium lines the upper part of the respiratory tract and functions to maintain airway integrity by providing both a physical barrier to inhaled noxious agents and a mechanism for their clearance via the mucociliary escalator. Ciliated columnar cells and goblet cells are the most important cell types in the normal respiratory epithelium. The other types of cells are represented by basal cells, brush cells and Kulchitsky cells (small granule cells). The normal architecture and function of airway epithelium is disturbed in chronic airway inflammatory diseases such as bronchial asthma. Airway remodeling is the general description for the thickening and restructuring of the airways seen in asthma patients. The characteristics of airway remodeling include inflammatory cell infiltration in lamina propria, subepithelial fibrosis, muscular and glandular hypertrophy, thickening of basement membrane and increased vascularity. Damage to the airway epithelium is one prominent feature of bronchial asthma. Epithelium damage includes gap openings, partial or total denudation, goblet cell metaplasia. The increased production of mucus can lead to the formation of plugs that contribute to airway obstruction. Mucin glycoproteins (MUC) are the major macromolecular component of mucus in normal airway epithelium. An increased expression of MUC2, MUC4 and MUC5B has been reported in asthmatic bronchial biopsies. At the epithelium level, in patients with bronchial asthma, appears an increased expression of Ki-67, p21 (WAF1) and decreased expression of FasL, Bcl-2 or Bax, too. Apoptosis of the airway epithelium is increasingly recognized as a potential mechanism by which damage may occur. More work is now needed to comprehend all aspects of this disease, including minimizing the ongoing damage to airway epithelium and consequent airway remodeling.

Keywords: Airway epithelium, bronchial asthma, epithelial lesions

1. Normal Respiratory Epithelium

The respiratory epithelium is a ciliated pseudostratified epithelium with goblet cells which line the airways, from the nasal cavities (except for the olfactory mucosa) to the intralobular bronchi (all the way to the entry in the pulmonary lobule) [1]. Scientifically, clinical terminology frequently uses the term "airway epithelium" while histology and histopathology use the term "respiratory epithelium". Because this text is founded on microscopic morphological information, characteristic for histology and histopathology, we opted to use "respiratory epithelium".

1.1. Characterization of the Respiratory Epithelium in Standard Light Microscopy

In standard light microscopy it appears as a heterogeneous mass of cells placed on a basement membrane, often thicker than for other epithelia with nuclei aligned at various levels. This characteristic led to the classification of the epithelium as a pseudostratified epithelium. In the structure of the respiratory epithelium one can easily notice, even in standard Hematoxylin-Eosin (HE) staining, the ciliated and goblet cells together with regenerative cells [2, 3].

Ciliated cells are tall columnar cells with acidophil cytoplasm and an ellipsoidal nucleus situated centrally or towards the basal domain. At the apical pole one can generally recognize cilia, which are numerous tapered expansions 7-10 μm in length and 0.25 μm in diameter (Figure 1). They normally float in the mucus on the surface of the epithelium produced by the goblet cells and the mucous glands in the wall of the airways [2, 4].

Goblet cells dispersed throughout the entire thickness of the respiratory epithelium are also tall columnar cells but smaller than the ciliated cells. In the apical 2/3 of the cell cytoplasm contains mucinogen granules with a merging tendency, making the staining with eosin very faint (Figure 1). The irregular, often triangular nucleus is pushed towards the basal domain of the cell. This microscopic aspect led to the comparison of the goblet cell with a "champagne glass" or with a "chalice flower" [2, 5]. Special stains such as mucicarmin, Alcian Blue or Periodic Acid Schiff (PAS) allow for easy identification of this type of cell by targeting the cytoplasmic mucus [4].

Goblet cells are not present in the structure of the respiratory epithelium at birth, appearing when the newborn is exposed to the external environment. Goblet cells are less numerous than ciliated cells, the ratio in the structure of the general respiratory epithelum being 1 goblet cell to 5 ciliated cells. Variations of this proportion can occur; the number of goblet cells may decrease towards the intralobular territory [5]. The exposure to a polluted environment (including second-hard smoke) leads to an increase in the number of goblet cells throughout the respiratory epithelium.

Renewal cells are cuboidal and can be identified by the alignment of rounded nuclei above the basement membrane [1, 2] (Figure 1).

1.2. Characterization of the Respiratory Epithelium in Electron Microscopy

Electron microscopy uncovers 6 types of cells in the structure of the respiratory epithelium. Alongside the three cell types depicted previously, there are cells with microvilli at their apical pole (type I and II) and endocrine cells (Kulchitsky cells) [2, 5].

In electron microscopy, ciliated cells have cell organelles common for any other cell, the only specificity being the presence at the apical pole of hundreds of vibrating cilia placed in concentric circles.

The cilia ensure the unidirectional displacement, by quick and synchronized movements, of mucus on the on the surface of the cell by which they remove large particles (3-5 μm) from inhaled air. This mechanism of filtration makes them a component of the muco-ciliated barrier. In the nasal cavities, the movement of the cilia is orientated towards the pharynx, while in the trachea it is orientated towards the larynx [6, 7].

Every cilium has a peripheral plasma membrane and an interior cytoskeleton named the axoneme. The axoneme consists of a complex of microtubules: a central pair (C1 and C2) around which 9 doublets of peripheral microtubules are uniformly arranged. The central pair is separated from the peripheral doublets by a discontinuous central sheath projection at 14-nm intervals along the length of the cilium. Every peripheral pair consists of an A-microtubule and a B-microtubule. Every microtubule has 13 protofilaments arranged helicoidally due to alternating polymerization of α tubulin and β tubulin. In the peripheral doublets the complete A-microtubule, consisting of 13 protofilaments, attaches an incomplete B-microtubule which consists of 10 protofilaments. On each A-microtubule there are dynein molecules (a protein with ATP activity) arranged as arms radiating towards the B-microtubule of the neighboring doublet, spaced at 24 nm intervals. Molecules of nexin, present at 86 nm intervals, play an important role in the attachment of an A-microtubule of one doublet to the B-microtubule of the following doublet. The connection between the central doublet and the peripheral one is achieved by radial spokes expanding from each peripheral doublet towards the central pair spaced at 29 nm intervals. At the base of the cilium, in the cell's apical domain, there is a basal body which is a structure similar to the centrosome and is considered as a modified centrosome [2, 4].

Goblet cells have at their enlarged apical pole a series of short microvilli; the basal pole is tapered and fixated on the basement membrane. In the apical two thirds of cell, the cytoplasm is occupied by secretory vacuoles containing mucus. In the basal third of cell we can find the nucleus along with the rest of the cytoplasmic organelles (SER, Golgi complex) [4, 8].

In electron microscopy the renewal cells in the structure of the respiratory epithelium are cuboidal cells which do not touch the surface of the epithelium. Their cytoplasm contains a small number of cell organelles [3].

Type I brush-border cells are tall columnar cells, impossible to differentiate in the epithelial cellular mass in light microscopy. In electron microscopy they have microvilli at their apical pole but in the cytoplasm there can be noted a small number of cell organelles except for mitochondria. At the basal pole, type I brush-border cells come into close proximity with sensitive axonal terminations and thus are considered as cells with a role in chemoreception in the respiratory epithelium [2, 5].

Type II brush-border cells have, like the type I cells, microvilli at their apical pole but they can be differentiated from the latter by better represented organelles, numerous basal corpuscles and the absence of contact with nervous terminations. Due to these characteristics they are believed to be immature ciliated cells [5, 8].

Kulchitsky cells, which appear either isolated or organized into small groups, are cuboidal cells. They are similar to renewal cells but in the cytoplasm there are a series of secretory granules, thus being called small granule cells. The granules have between 100 and 300 nm diameter, are lined by a membrane and have an electron-dense core surrounded by a more transparent halo. The immunocytochemistry techniques proved that these cells produce various polypeptides with endocrine and paracrine activity (serotonin, encephalin, endorphins, calcitonin, bombesin). Consequently, they were classified as enteroendocrine cells. Their number is highest at birth and decreases progressively with aging. Their presence explains the possibility of carcinoid tumors occurring at this level [2].

The cells are consolidated in the epithelium by a series of cell junctions called desmosomes. The desmosomes (*macula adherens*) are junctions between two epithelial cells with the shape of oval discoid structures with a long axis of 400-500 nm and a short axis of 100 nm.

In electron microscopy, the structure of the desmosome is centered by an intercellular space of approximately 30 nm, in the middle of which appears a discrete electron-dense line. On either side of the electron-dense line, the cytoplasm adjacent to the inner face of the plasmalema contains a dense area called an "attachment plaque" or a "desmosomal plaque" (400 x 250 x 10 nm).

Towards these dense areas, intermediate filaments converge. The main molecules in the intercellular space are represented by desmoglein 1, desmocolin 1 and desmocolin 2, which is a part of the cadherin superfamily. In the desmosome plaque there are unglycosylated attachment proteins: desmoplakin 1, desmoplakin 2, plakoglobin, desmiokin or a basic polypeptide. These molecules establish links with intermediate cytokeratin filaments within the cytoplasm of the epithelial cells which insert into the plaque and come out again in a "hairpin-like" trajectory [4, 7, 8].

Alongside adherent junctions there are also cummunication junctions (gap junctions), which allow selective intercellular diffusion of ions and small molecules. In electron microscopy, in the territory of communication junctions a small space (3 nm) is noticed because the cells are not joined directly with their plasma membranes. In this space there are described severeal bridge-like structures passing from one cell to the other, called connexons. Connexons have a tubular arrangement (with a central space) through which ions and small molecules such as cyclic AMP, some hormones or aminoacids can pass.

This is similar to two cells which are joined and form a channel with a 2 nm diameter [4, 8].

In association with these cell types, characteristic for respiratory epithelium, in some areas of the respiratory airways there can be found M cells which are epithelial cells associated with lymphoid tissue which differentiate during organogenesis (in the digestive epithelium as well).

The M cell is also called an “en dome” cell due to its peculiar bell shape, with short irregular microvilli at the apical pole. This cell functions as a transport pathway for antigen structures (and not as an antigen-presenting cell). Without intracellular modification, they are released through the basal pole into the space created by the bell-shape of the cell. After transport, antigens are engulfed by macrophages or intraepithelial lymphocytes or can completely cross the surface epithelium reaching the *lamina propria* [5].

1.3. The Relationship between the Respiratory Epithelium and the Basement Membrane

Between the surface epithelium and the subjacent connective tissue there is a special structure called the basement membrane. For the respiratory epithelium the basement membrane is thicker than in other places. It can be readily observed in standard light microscopy due to special stains: PAS (staining burgundy red) or argentic impregnation (it colors in brownish-black) (Figure 2) [3, 8].

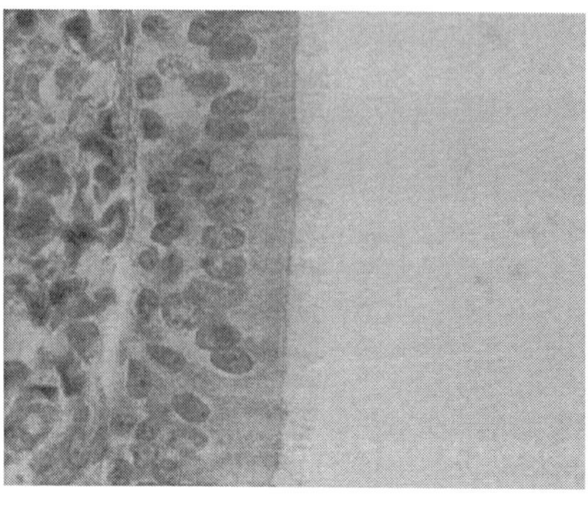

Figure 1. Normal respiratory epithelium (trichrome Szekelly, x 400).

In electron microscopy, the basement membrane of the respiratory epithelium respects the complex organization of all basement membranes, consisting of three laminas: *lamina lucida*, *lamina densa* and *lamina reticularis*. *Lamina lucida* and *lamina densa* together form the basal lamina. The basal lamina is synthetized by the surface epithelium. *Lamina reticularis* is produced by the connective tissue [4]. *Lamina lucida* is transparent in electron microscopy, being 45 nm thick. One can observe moderate condensations in hemidesmosome territories.

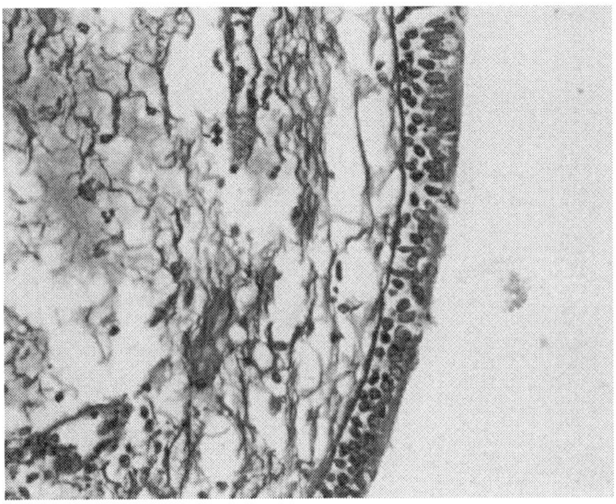

Figure 2. Normal basement membrane (Gordon Sweet, x 200).

Through biochemistry, at this level, a series of glycoproteins were identified, such as: laminin, entactin, basement membrane glycoprotein as well as transmembranary proteins from the family of the integrins which project from the epithelial cell membrane towards the basal lamina [2, 4]. *Lamina densa* is an electron-dense area, 50 nm thick.

Through biochemistry it was determined that it consists of protein molecules: laminin and type IV collagen arranged in a "wire fence" pattern surrounded by proteoglycans such as perlecan, fibronectin, type V collagen, adhesion molecules from the family of integrins [2, 4]. *Lamina reticularis* is formed by type I and III collagen. It is placed between the basal lamina and the subjacent connective tissue, its thickness being variable according to the forces exerted on the surface epithelium [2, 4].

Electron microscopy showed that all the cells of the respiratory epithelium, even if of various heights, come in direct contact with the basement membrane. Consequently, the respiratory epithelium can be considered a simple epithelium. If the fixation of the cells within the epithelium is achieved by intercellular desmosomal type junctions, their anchorage on the basement membrane is realized through hemidesmosomal junctions [3, 4].

In electron microscopy, the hemidesmosome has a similar structure to the above described desmosome having an intracellular attachment plaque in the cytoplasm adjacent to the cell membrane of the basal pole. Biochemically, the attachment plaque consists of proteins from the desmoplakin-like family (plectin, BP 230 and erbin), able to secure cytokeratin intermediate filaments which do not reenter the cytoplasm after entering the plaque.

Thus, the U-shape trajectory characteristic for the desmosomes is absent. Transmembranar molecules such as calcium-dependent cadherins, present in the structure of the desmosomes, are replaced by integrins (α4β6 integrin) or similar molecules (type XVII collagen, CD151 glycoprotein) acting as matrix-cells receptors which ensure the attachment to the laminin and type IV collagen in the structure of the basement membrane [4, 7, 8].

1.4. Lamina Propria

The respiratory epithelium is placed on a connective tissue sheet called the *lamina propria* [1]. This is a loose connective tissue with a rich blood and nerve supply, with many elastic fibers, along with fixed (fibroblasts, fibrocytes) and free cells (macrophages, mast cells, plasma cells, lymphocytes).

An increased number of migrated cells determine the classification of this type of connective tissue as a "defense chorion" together with the one in the digestive tube [5]. The increased number of lymphocytes in the wall of the big respiratory airways explains the possibility of lymphoid infiltrations or even of lymphoid nodules occurrence – components of BALT (bronchus-associated lymphoid tissue) [5].

Lamina propria also contains tubulo-acinous sero-mucous glands (Bowman's glands) consisting of acini and short excretion ducts lined by a simple cuboidal epithelium allowing the release of secretion products on the surface of the epithelium [5].

2. Fibrobronchoscopy in Asthma: Pros and Cons

Fibrobronchoscopy represents the most adequate evaluation method of airway modifications in asthma because it allows a direct visualization of the large airways and a bronchoalveolar lavage and/or a bronchial biopsy. Nevertheless, the procedure is invasive and therefore rarely accepted by asthma patients with respiratory insufficiency. Although the scientific impact of its results, leading to further research in the pathogeny of asthma, is uncontestable, fibrobronchoscopy accompanied or not by a biopsy is not a routine exam in asthma. Within the context of asthmatic pathology, the fibronchoscopy investigation is practiced mainly with research purposes, fact supported by a relatively small number of publications in literature (approximately 200 in 20 years) [9]. According to the literature, microscopic exams of bronchial mucosa fragments harvested through fibrobronchoscopy obviously opens new perspectives for deciphering physiopathology in asthma. In order to minimalize the risk of an incomplete harvest it is recommended to obtain 5 to 7 fragments of bronchial mucosa *via* a biopsy for each patient examined through fibrobronchoscopy [9].

Because the investigated patients may have bronchial obstruction in varying degrees, fibrobronchoscopy calls for a series of supplementary safety measures (careful supervision of patients, the administration of bronchodilators in the same day as the investigation, supplementation of oxygen therapy during the exam) in order to prevent the risk of complications (decrease of oxygen saturation [10, 11], cough, wheezing [12].

A pioneering study in fibrobronchoscopy [13] states that a biopsy combined with lavage can be performed on asthma patients but it demands supplementary caution on patients with increased bronchial reactivity. The explanation is the significant decrease in Forced Expiratory Volume 1 (FEV1) recorded in asthmatic as well as in healthy patients [13]. The decrease in FEV1 is inversely correlated with the quantity of methacholine necessary to reduce FEV1 by 20% compared to values previous to fibrobronchoscopy but it cannot be correlated with the score for the symptoms, the usage of inhaled beta2-agonists and with the variations of Peak Expiratory Flow (PEF) recorded in the 2 weeks preceding the exam. Moreover, the authors report a significant decrease in oxygen saturation during the biopsy (an average of 3% with variations between -1 and 17%) without correlation with severity indexes in asthma [13].

Our research focused on the pathology of asthma which was made possible by the close cooperation with the staff of The Clinical Pneumology Hospital in Iaşi. The experience of the staff in the performance of fibrobronchoscopy with bronchial biopsy in asthma patients with varying degrees of the disease's severity confirmed the presence of desaturation in severe forms of the illness and its absence in moderate and milder forms (intermittent and slightly persistent asthma). For the patients investigated on our joint research the most important decrease of oxygen saturation was 10% (from 90% to 80%) the average recorded value being 1.3%.

The evaluation of the clinical (score of the symptoms), paraclinical (arterial saturation, PEF) and therapeutic (usage of inhaled beta2-agonists) parameters consequent to the fibrobronchoscopy reveals the absence of a direct relationship between the invasiveness of the procedure and the evolution of the disease [14]. The degree of arterial O_2 saturation and the decrease in PEF were similar for asthmatic and healthy patients. Nevertheless, the decrease in PEF and bronchial hyperreactivity were significantly reduced in the bronchial biopsy by comparison with the situation where the biopsy was associated with bronchoalveolar lavage [14].

The research dedicated to the advantages and disadvantages, to the limits and the risks of this diagnosis technique allowed the revision of the initial guidelines, recommending the fibrobronchoscopy with biopsy and lavage including for the patients with more severe obstruction (FEV1 $< 60\%$) [15]. There is data supporting the statement that bronchial biopsy is well tolerated even by asthma patients who did not receive bronchodilating medication [11]. This conduct should be avoided due to the risk of a much more severe obstruction occurring after bronchoscopy. According to a meta-analysis [16], including 6 independent studies on the safety of the technique bronchoscopy, endobronchial biopsy and bronchoalveolar lavage, these can be applied on asthma patients with different degrees of severity. The most complications arise when both harvesting procedures are practiced, lavage as well as biopsy, which leads to the conclusion that bronchoalveolar lavage is responsible in most cases for the reported adverse effects.

The results of our interdisciplinary research team are based on a bronchoscopic examination performed in complete safety, in a controlled environment, without unpredicted events or secondary effects leading to a possible interruption of the exam. None of the patients presented an exacerbation of the disease in the days following the fibrobronchoscopy and did not require systemic corticotherapy or the increase of the dosage in corticotherapy.

3. Epithelial Lesions in Asthma

The bronchial mucosa fragments, harvested through fibrobronchoscopy, were routinely processed for HE and other special stains.

The microscopic exam in HE stain is mandatory as the first stage towards the evaluation of the quality of the harvested fragments in order to confirm the possibility of interpretation of the lesions. Thus, it is necessary the existence of the epithelium and of a subepithelial connective sheet of minimum 0.3 mm and the quality of the fixation and coloration has to be also appraised. The analysis of a bronchial biopsy is affected by the presence of tissue fragmentation, pieces of hyaline cartilage, extended hemorrhage or large quantities of mucus.

In the bronchial biopsies harvested from asthma patients the most important modifications are in the epithelium such as epithelial desquamation, hyperplasia of goblet cells and squamous epithelial metaplasia.

3.1. Epithelial Desquamation

Frequently, the respiratory epithelium presents partial epithelial desquamation lesions with the preservation of a "basal" layer of cells on the basement membrane or areas of complete desquamation with complete exposure of the basement membrane. In favor of the idea that epithelial desquamation (complete or partial) could represent a lesion marker in asthma, the following can be observed:

- bronchial epithelial desquamation lesions were noticed both from tissue fragments harvested postmortem from patients deceased after an acute asthma attack and from those obtained through endoscopy from patients with stable chronic asthma [17, 18];
- the presence of "Creola" bodies in the sputum of asthma patients [19];
- the presence of an increased number of epithelial cells in the bronchoalveolar lavage liquid in patients with asthma [20], in which the number of shed cells were directly correlated with the degree of bronchial hyperreactivity [21].

Nevertheless, numerous studies in literature support the idea that bronchial epithelial desquamation in asthma represents in fact an artifact of harvest, processing and inclusion of tissue fragments obtained through endoscopy and not a characteristic morphologic lesion [22]. The idea is founded on the conclusions of various research performed on large groups of volunteer patients as opposed to groups of asthma patients.

Thus, partial or complete epithelial desquamation was also identified in fragments of bronchial mucosa harvested from healthy patients [23, 24]. Cell composition of sputum and of the bronchoalveolar lavage liquid was identical for the control and asthma patients [23]. The degree and spread of epithelial desquamation are not statistically significant correlated with values of FEV1 [24]. Some specialists explain the presence of an increased number of epithelial cells in the bronchoalveolar lavage liquid in patients with asthma by the fact that the harvesting procedure represents a direct trauma on an already fragile epithelium [21].

Data in literature [25] reconfirms the role of the epithelial junctions by indicating the preservation of only one cell layer depleted of ciliated or goblet cells (interpreted as partial denudation) on 50% of the length of the analyzed fragments and complete denudation of the basement membrane on 10 to 15% of the length of the same fragments. Partial denudation on larger areas versus complete denudation on smaller areas can also be explained by the fact that desmosome junctions are easier to damage than junctions between epithelial cells and the basement membrane such as hemidesmosomes which are associated with adhesion molecules like integrins and anchorage filaments [25]. Within the same context, recent research shows that beta 4 integrin, a molecule ensuring the adhesion of epithelial cells in normal respiratory epithelium, has a decreased expression in asthma patients. This molecular modification could explain the perturbation of epithelial cell homeostasis in asthma patients [26].

These controversial opinions on epithelial desquamation have an important reflection on the theory according to which the loss of epithelial barrier may favor bronchial hyperreactivity in asthmatic patients. The classic theory is replaced by a new one, focused on the intact epithelium acting as a "proinflammatory organ" directly intervening in reshaping of bronchial wall [27, 28].

The research of our team on epithelial modifications associated with asthma revealed partial or complete epithelial desquamation of the bronchial epithelium. The areas of partial epithelial desquamation were present both in healthy and in almost all asthma patients (94.73%). Complete epithelial desquamation was not noticed on bronchial biopsies harvested from control patients but it was present in 55.26% of the asthma patients regardless of the severity of the disease (Figure 3, 4).

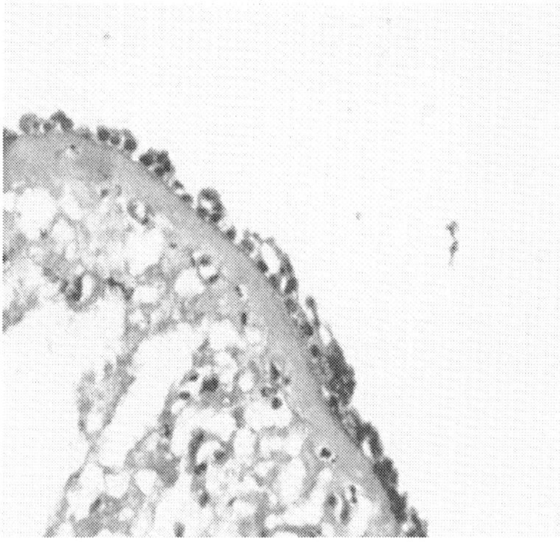

Figure 3. Partial epithelial desquamation – mild persistent asthma (HE, x 100).

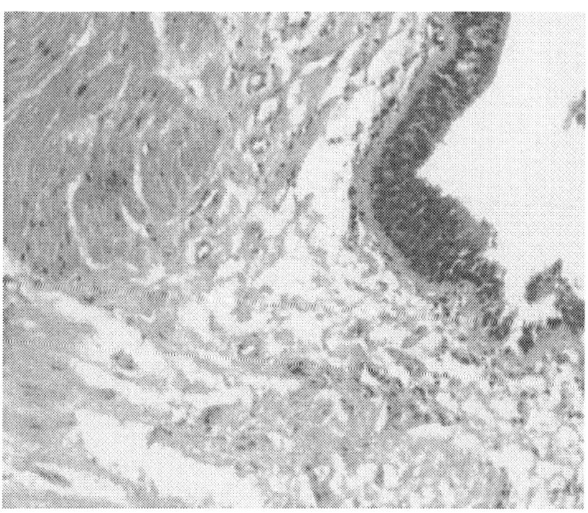

Figure 4. Partial epithelial desquamation associated with a complete epithelial desquamation area – moderate persistent asthma (HE, x 100).

Our results support the statement that although these lesions are frequently observed in the microscopic exam they are not specific for asthma. Epithelial desquamation may also occur in other respiratory pathologies and their presence is not significantly correlated with the severity of the disease.

3.2. Hyperplasia of Goblet Cells

In the bronchial mucosa, mucus secretion has two points of origin: one from goblet cells of the epithelium and the other from glandular mucous cells. Normal mucus secretion vary between 10 and 100 ml/24 hours and is 96% water, the rest represented by electrolytes, lipids, amino acids, immunoglobulins, albumins and enzymes [8, 29]. The mucus layer [29, 30] consists of two layers: an inferior one, 5 μm thick, and a superior one, 1-2 μm thick. The inferior layer has a relatively more watery consistency and ensures the movement of the cilia. The upper layer has a greater mucous consistency and comes in contact only with the tips of the cilia.

Normally the mucus layer continuously moves towards the pharynx where it is swallowed with a speed of 1 cm per minute due to the effect of the cilia's movement. The cilia's movement is coordinated, and this phenomenon is called metachronism. Coughs and sneezes associated with muco-ciliary activity ensure the elimination of mucous secretions through air and digestive pathways (by deglutition) [29, 30].

Literature does not mention the development of the glandular area in bronchial mucosa fragments harvested from patients with intermittent and slightly persistent forms of asthma. Consequently, the increased mucus secretion is caused by goblet cell hyperplasia [31], which is a lesion with a constant frequency and a variable severity [31, 32].

One must note that the occurrence of a large number of goblet cells in the respiratory epithelial structure is not characteristic in asthma. This occurrence is a "response" of the epithelium to toxins such as tobacco smoke, to irritating particles in the environment and microorganisms [33, 34].

Although hyperplasia of goblet cells is reported even in the less severe stages of the disease, there are opposing opinions [35] based on studies with a work methodology which does not solidly support the conclusions (the identification of goblet cells being performed in standard coloration HE and the quantification through a semi-quantitative method). An extremely interesting study [36] indicates an increased number of goblet cells in asthma patients (93.043 ± 15.82) as opposed to healthy patients (41.95 ± 9.23) without size variations from one group to another. The level of mucin deposition was three times bigger in asthma patients as opposed to healthy patients. There were no differences in the levels of mucin deposition between patients with slightly persistent asthma and those with moderately persistent asthma, except that the levels of mucin secretion were significantly lower. According to this data, slightly persistent asthma is associated with hyperplasia of goblet cells with an increase in mucus deposits from the epithelium while in moderate cases of the disease there is an increase in the deposits as well as mucus secretion. These elements suggest the fact that the acute degranulation phenomenon of the goblet cells could represent the mechanism of symptom exacerbation in mild and moderate forms of asthma and chronic degranulation could contribute to the thickening of the bronchial wall in moderately persistent asthma [36].

The research of our team revealed the presence of hyperplasia lesions in goblet cells even on standard HE coloration. In order to quantify more precisely the degree of these lesions we performed an assessment of the extension of these modifications in the structure of the respiratory epithelium in asthma patients with different degrees of severity through the microscopic examination of specimens stained using the PAS technique (Figure 5, 6). Thus, we could observe the hyperplasic lesions of the goblet cells even in the early stages of the disease (intermittent asthma), with an increasing intensity showing a decrease in the FEV1 values.

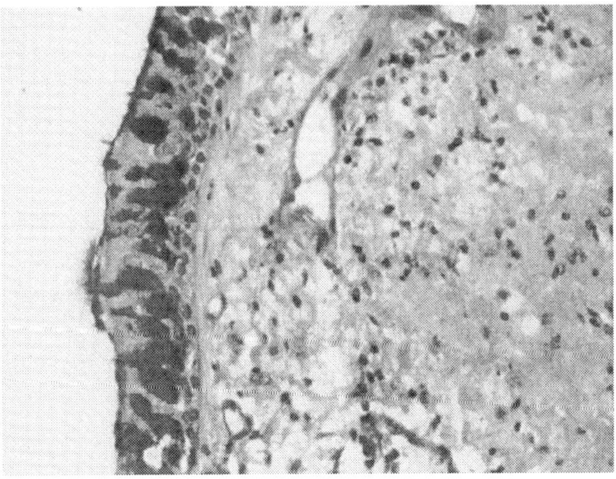

Figure 5. Moderately hyperplasia of goblet cells – mild persistent asthma (PAS, x 200).

Current research on the physiopathology of bronchial hypersecretion of mucus as well as on the mechanism of goblet cell hyperplasia is focused on several molecules involved either in regulation of mucus exocytosis (such as MARCKS – Myristoylated Alanine-Rich C Kinase) or in the increase of goblet cells numbers (such as EGF - Epidermal Growth Factor and CLCA - Calcium Activated Chloride Channels) or in the preservation of a large number of goblet cells (apoptotic factors Bcl-2 and Bax) [33]. Within the same context of the pathogenic mechanisms of asthma, experimental studies proved that there is an increase in the expression of some mucigen genes [22, 32, 37].

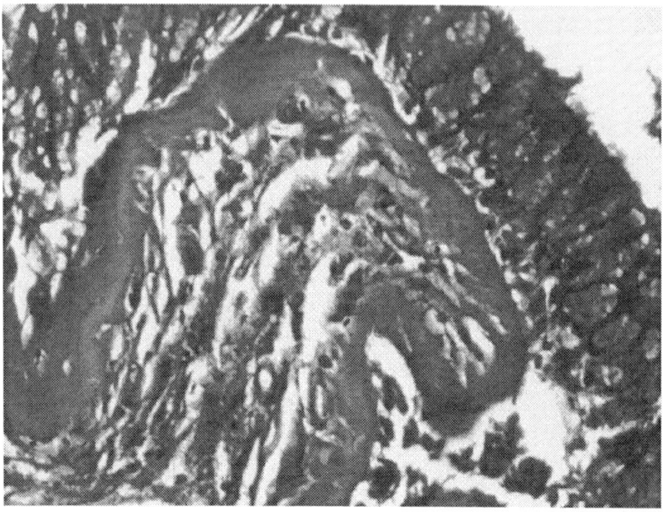

Figure 6. Important hyperplasia of goblet cells – moderate persistent asthma (PAS, x 200).

In humans there were described 20 MUC genes (genes that produce membrane-associated mucins), of which 9 are also expressed in the respiratory tract (MUC1, MUC2, MUC4, MUC5AC, MUC5B, MUC7, MUC8, MUC11 and MUC13). Recent research showed that normally, the genes coding MUC1, MUC2 and MUC8 are expressed in the respiratory epithelium as well as in submucosal glands, while MUC5AC and MUC13 are expressed only in the respiratory epithelium [38, 39]. Later, through immunohistochemistry (IHC), MUC5AC was identified in goblet cells and MUC5B and MUC7 were exclusively at the glandular level [40]. Interestingly, ciliated cells of the respiratory epithelium express MUC4 [40].

This distribution of MUC gene expression in the respiratory tract changes in pathological conditions characterized by mucus hypersecretion such as asthma. Most studies in literature support an increase in MUC5AC, MUC 2 and MUC4 gene expression in asthma patients with varying degrees of severity of the disease [36, 37, 41].

On the other hand, deceased patients with asthma present a significant expression of the MUC5B gene [42, 43]. This sustains the implication of submucosa glands in the hypersecretion of mucus in these patients [42, 43]. This observation raises the importance of the primary involvement of goblet cells.

Mucus hypersecretion remains an important morbidity and mortality factor in pulmonary pathology (including asthma). The possibility of controlling the mucus quantity in the respiratory pathways focuses on the inhibition of nerve activity (by tachikinic receptor antagonists) or the inhibition of mucin exocytosis (through Munc-18B blockers). Other possible therapeutic methods are based on mucin synthesis and goblet cell hyperplasia inhibition (through EGF inhibitors and tyrosin-kinase receptor inhibitors) or the control of goblet cells apoptosis (inductor Bax molecules or Bcl-2 inhibitors) [44]. The latter aspect is also supported by recent research on lab animals, according to which the resolution of goblet cell allergen induced hyperplasia is controlled by γ-interferon through Bax [45].

3.3. Epithelial Metaplasia

Epithelial metaplasia, described in literature as a possible manifestation of the respiratory epithelium subjected to a chronic inflammatory aggression [31, 46], was identified in our research performed on 38 asthmatic patients in 16 cases, 4 with a mild form, 7 with moderate persistent form and 3 diagnosed with severe persistent asthma. We must emphasis the fact that we excluded from our study groups smokers, because they constantly present epithelial transformations secondary to the chronic exposure to substances in cigarette smoke.

3.4. Epithelial Proliferative Activity

In response to the chronic aggression expressed in the morphology by an increased fragility, leading to cell desquamation the respiratory epithelium, will react in order to reestablish its integrity through two fundamental mechanisms: either an increase in cell proliferation in order to replace the injured cells or an extension of cell survival through the inhibition of the factors controlling programmed cellular death (apoptosis). It appears that both processes coexist in the respiratory epithelium affected by asthma.

Consequently, numerous studies in literature focused on the transformations in the expression of cell proliferation factors (Ki-67, PCNA) as well as that of apoptosis factors in the respiratory epithelium in patients with varying degrees of severity and also by comparison with normal respiratory epithelium. Data in literature reveals the fact that the aggression exerted by several allergens leads to an increase in the proliferative activity of the respiratory epithelium in intermittent and slightly persistent asthma [46] and also that there appears to be a direct relationship between the levels of PCNA expression and the thickness of the respiratory epithelium [47].

The comparative examination [48] of three groups (control, asthma patients with or without corticosteroid treatment) revealed that the respiratory epithelium of patients under treatment express at the same time Bcl-2, Fas, FasL and PCNA. The authors conclude that steroid treatment applied to patients with asthma leads to a decrease in the inflammation of the bronchial wall (especially the eosinophil one) and it promotes cell survival and proliferation, possibly due to the influence on the expression of Bcl-2 and PCNA [48]. However, corticosteroid treatment applied chronically to asthma patients does not succeed to control the balance between the proliferation and cell death in the respiratory epithelium. As a result, the attempt to reestablish epithelial integrity fails. The alteration of epithelial structural integrity constitutes a key element in the pathologic mechanism by which the disease maintains itself [49]. Consequently, epithelial dysfunction contributes on a morphological level to the structural reshaping of the bronchial wall and on a functional level to the decline of pulmonary functions. Therefore, recent opinions support the necessity of new therapeutic targets in asthma focusing on the control of the epithelial proliferation even more so due to the fact that the steroid treatment proved to be inefficient [49].

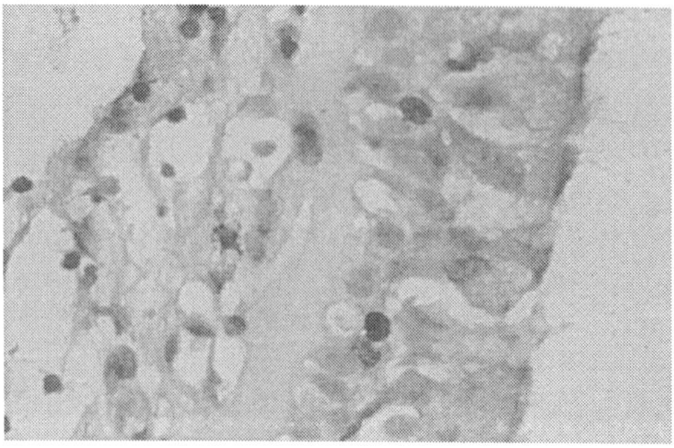

Figure 7. A small number of Ki-67-positive cells in bronchial epithelium – intermittent asthma (IHC, anti-Ki-67, x 400).

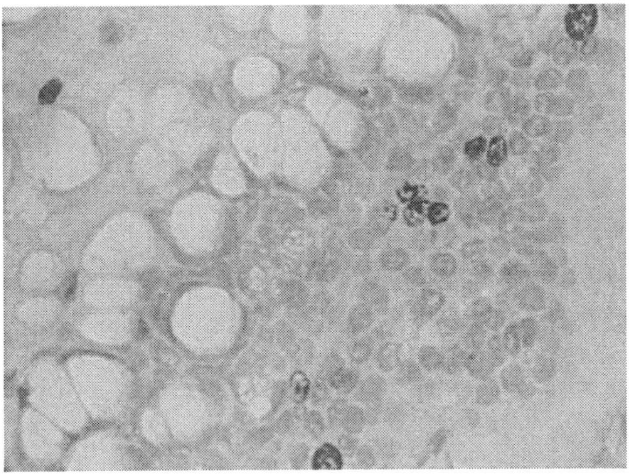

Figure 8. Ki-67-positive cells forming small clusters in bronchial epithelium – severe persistent asthma (IHC, anti-Ki-67, x 400).

In our research, directed to the evaluation of proliferative activity, we determined an increase in the level of Ki-67 expression (corresponding to the proliferation rate) in the respiratory epithelium in asthma patients as compared to the control patients. Nevertheless, the bronchial epithelium did not prove to be hyperproliferative [50]. Ki-67-positive cells were present sporadically near the basement membrane along the epithelium in milder forms and reached a maximum as number and a clustering tendency in severely persistent forms of asthma (Figure 7, 8) [50].

The statistical analysis revealed the existence of a statistically significant correlation between the number of Ki-67 positive cells and the severity of the disease ($r=0.887$, $p \ll 0.01$, 95% CI) [50].

3.5. Epithelial Apoptosis

Apoptosis, defined as programmed cell death, constitutes a normal sequence in tissue development, morphogenesis and equilibrium. In the context of regulation deficiencies, causing perturbations in the DNA repair mechanism and the modification of the cell cycle, apoptosis contributes to the establishment of pathologic conditions. Apoptosis is a multiple-factor phenomenon produced by the specific activation of an intracellular cysteine proteinase family named caspases [51]. The apoptotic process can be achieved two different ways. The intrinsic path (mitochondrial path, type I) is regulated by apoptotic protein members of the Bcl-2 family and by specific caspases through the implication of the mitochondria which release proteins activating the caspases in the cytosol thus triggering apoptosis [52]. The extrinsic path (transmembranar path, type II) is regulated by Fas proteins and by the proteins of the tumor necrosis factor receptor (TNF-R), involving specific caspases inducing apoptosis by linking the ligand to the cell surface [53]. The molecular family Bcl-2 includes members which by promoting cell survival are believed to be anti-apoptotic (Bcl-2, Bcl-X_L), together with members coordinating cell death, considered as pro-apoptotic (Bax, Bak). The Bax molecule, initially identified by immunoprecipitation as the link partner for Bcl-2 [54] has a physiological role in the embryonic development as it is overexpressed as a response to the presence of apoptotic stimuli.

Most studies in the literature support the existence of a growing proliferation rate in injured respiratory epithelium even in the early stages of the disease. Not the same can be stated about the aspects regarding the level and control of apoptosis as the second mechanism through which epithelial integrity can be restored. This is mainly due to the fact that, currently, there is little information with regard to the level and the control mechanism behind programmed cell death in normal respiratory epithelium [55]; obtaining fragments of normal bronchial mucosa through a fibrobronchoscopy examination is difficult. The apoptotic process in the respiratory epithelial cells is absolutely normal and necessary because the cell number can be controlled and lesions secondary to viral infections or allergen induced can be limited. In literature there are data referring to the apoptosis of ciliated and goblet cells in normal bronchial epithelium [56] but none regarding the apoptosis of renewal cells. Research on respiratory epithelium apoptosis in a normal and a pathologic context (including asthma) is oriented on the anti and pro-apoptotic intervention of members of the Bcl-2 family [49, 55, 57, 58]. Studies on the respiratory epithelium in asthma reveal an increase of epithelial cell apoptosis through the different interventions of anti and pro-apoptotic factors. In the category of inductors we include, besides allergen substances, the elements in cigarette smoke, some cytokines (TGF-1), infectious agents (viruses and bacteria) and hypoxia [55, 57]. Sadly, due to the large variability of asthma, the extreme diversity of the study groups and the differences in the interpretations of the immunohistochemistry exams, data regarding the expression of the anti-apoptotic factor Bcl-2 in the respiratory epithelium in asthma are controversial. Moreover, current studies in literature, referring to the level of the pro-apoptotic expression of Bax in the respiratory epithelium in asthma patients, are very scarce.

- Anti-apoptosis activity – the expression of Bcl-2

Some studies demonstrate an increase of Bcl-2 expression in the bronchial epithelium in asthma patients in comparison with control patients [48, 59], mainly in the renewal basal layer and directly correlated with steroid treatment [48], suggesting that anti-apoptosis represents a self-protection mechanism in chronic inflammatory aggression [59]. However, these studies are contradicted by more recent investigations noting a decrease in the expression of the Bcl-2 factor in the respiratory epithelium especially for the patients with severely persistent forms by comparison with the milder forms of asthma [49, 55].

Our results [60] support these latest findings because in the group we investigated we noted a significant decrease in the expression of the Bcl-2 factor in patients with severely persistent asthma as opposed to patients diagnosed with milder forms of the disease and in control patients (Figure 9, 10).

The statistical analysis revealed the existence of a significant inverse correlation between the severity of asthma (expressed through the FEV1) and the levels of Bcl-2 expression ($r = -0.7349$, $p<<0.01$, 95%CI). Pertaining to location, the immunohistochemical positive cells were mostly observed in the basal layer of the respiratory epithelium, except for the squamous metaplasia areas, where Bcl-2 positive cells could be found in the superficial layers too.

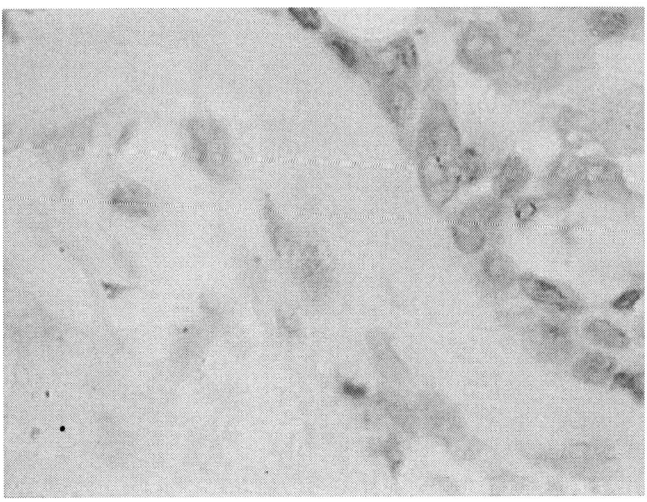

Figure 9. Moderately positive reaction (++) at the bronchial epithelium level – mild ersistent asthma (IHC, anti-Bcl-2, x 600).

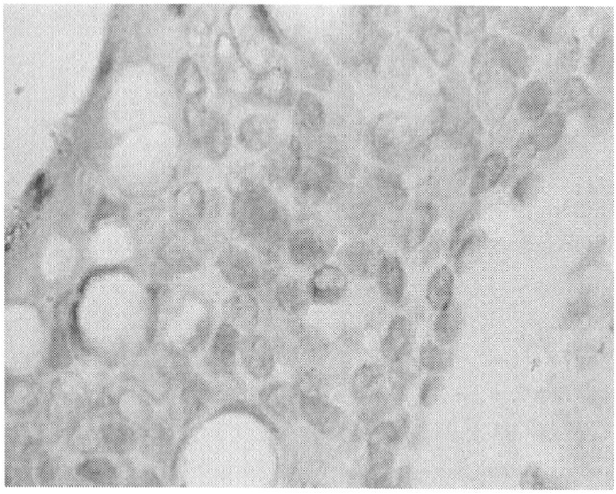

Figure 10. Slightly positive reaction (+) at the bronchial epithelium level – severe persistent asthma (IHC, anti-Bcl-2, x 600).

- Pro-apoptotic activity – the expression of Bax

The investigation of Bax expression in the respiratory epithelium, harvested post-mortem from asthma patients with varying degrees of severity by comparison with the normal respiratory epithelium, revealed a decrease in the expression of Bax in all asthma patients (even in milder stages of the disease) as opposed to control patients [61]. These observations are also supported by several studies showing a decrease in the number of goblet cells under the influence of γ-interferon, a substance which contributes to the activation of the pro-apoptosis factor Bax [62, 63]. Our research [60], confirmed by statistical analysis, showed a decrease of Bax expression in the bronchial epithelium of all asthma patients in comparison with the control patients even in the intermittent asthma stage ($r=-0.617$, $p=0.0265$, 95%CI). The statistical study performed outlined the absence of a significant association between the degree of severity in asthma and the level of Bax expression ($\chi^2=1.77$, $p=0.6206$, 95%CI) [60]. We must stress the fact that Bax-positive cells were observed "focally" in the structure of the respiratory epithelium, these being present in territories with various lesions such as epithelium denudation or squamous metaplasia (Figure 11, 12). Thus, today it is believed that the decrease in Bax expression levels at the level of the respiratory epithelium in asthma patients even in the early stages of the disease is an element supporting the prolongation of goblet cell life in its structure and the hypersecretion of mucus [44].

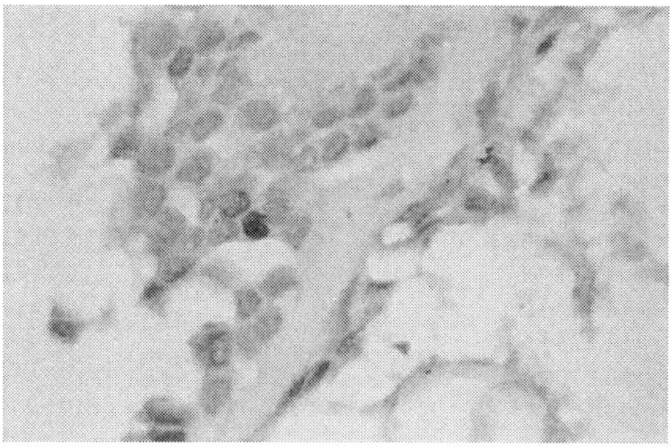

Figure 11. Slightly positive reaction (+) at the bronchial epithelium level – intermittent asthma (IHC, anti-Bax, x 600).

Consequently, the identification of a controlled "regulation" for the Bax expression in the respiratory epithelium represents a new research direction, with a benefic effect in the treatment of mucus hypersecretion in asthma. The issue of apoptosis in respiratory epithelium cells in asthma patients still remains open especially because more and more authors, on the basis of their own research, bring into discussion once again the theory according to which the steroid treatment itself (especially in the larger dosage used in patients with severe forms of the disease) would constitute a factor in increased apoptosis of respiratory epithelium in asthma patients [55, 64, 65, 66, 67].

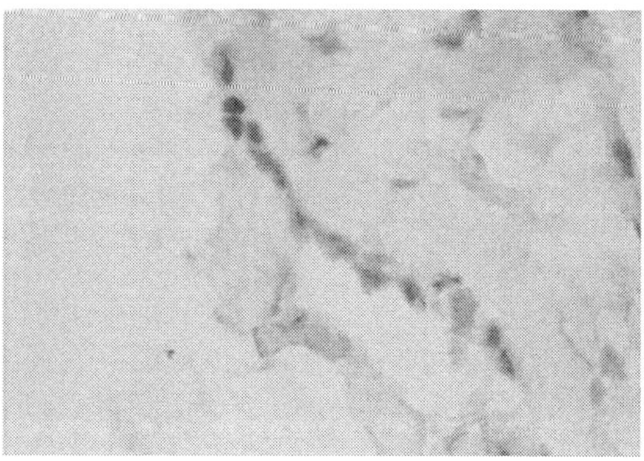

Figure 12. Slightly positive reaction (+) at the bronchial epithelium level – severe persistent asthma (IHC, anti-Bax, x 600).

- Other factors involved in apoptosis

Recent studies showed that Zn has an anti-apoptotic role, intervening through the inhibition of caspases associated with antioxidant activity and cell membrane stabilization [68]. The correlation of this observation with the decreased levels of Zn in chronic inflammatory diseases of the respiratory tract [69] lead to promoting and administrating Zn supplements as a protection factor toward the occurrence of lesions in respiratory epithelial cells [70].

The molecule p21 (Cip1/WAF1), kinase-dependent cyclin inhibitor, intervenes in the regulation of cell proliferation and death [71, 72]. Studies performed on human subjects [73] along with experimental studies (using genetically modified rats with the absence of p21 gene) [73] showed an increase of p21 expression in the respiratory epithelium of asthma patients and consequently an intensification of apoptosis unlike in the control group. The manipulation of p21 expression could represent another new therapeutic target in asthma even more so because the expression of p21 is not influenced by corticosteroid treatment [74].

Another two investigated molecules in the context of the relationship between cigarette smoke and apoptosis are peroxiredoxin V (PRXV), a protein with antioxidant potential [75], and pirin, intensely expressed and associated with the stimulation of apoptosis [76].

Conclusion

Although fibrobronchoscopy is not a current diagnostic method, it allowed the acquirement of bronchial mucosa fragments from patients diagnosed with different stages of asthma. Thus, we were able to describe the epithelial lesions and those of the bronchial wall even from the stages of intermittent and slightly persistent asthma, fact which was not possible until now because bronchial mucosa fragments were harvested only during autopsies in deceased patients due to severe asthma crises. The possibility of analyzing bronchial mucosa fragments represented the "starting point" for research on morphologic, physio-pathological and clinical correlations in asthma.

Current existing data is still insufficient mainly because of the difficulties in acquiring bronchial mucosa fragments. The use of fibrobronchoscopy in asthma is limited. Furthermore, the great variability of the disease and different methodologies used according to different laboratories may influence the interpretation of the final results of microscopic and immunohistochemical exams.

Important steps were recorded in the deciphering of the lesions in the respiratory epithelium injured by asthma. Besides the descriptive characterization of microscopic lesions in the respiratory epithelium, the increase in the Ki-67 cell proliferation factor expression and the decrease in the expression of anti-apoptosis factor Bcl-2 support the idea of the so-called "reparatory phenotype" of the epithelium. We do not have all the answers for all the questions regarding the factors or the mechanisms leading to the collapse of these structural repair processes in the epithelium. Most opinions support the role of the chronic injury of the epithelium sustaining the inflammatory process in the bronchial wall which exerts a new aggressive action on the already injured epithelium. Current research in asthma involve molecular and cellular biology aspects, with a direct orientation on the intervention and action mechanism of growth and repair factors and also of pro and anti-apoptotic factors.

The final purpose is not just to reach an understanding of the intimate pathologic mechanisms taking place in the epithelium and in the entire bronchial wall in asthma, but to also discover new therapeutic modalities in order to control asthmatic phenomenon and to improve the life quality in asthma patients.

References

[1] Fawcett, DW; Jensh, RP. *Bloom and Fawcett's Concise Histology*, 2nd ed. London: Arnold; 2002.

[2] Ross, MH; Pawlina, W. *Histology. A Text and Atlas with Correlated Cell and Molecular Biology*, 6th ed. Philadelphia: Lippincott Williams and Wilkins; 2010.

[3] Ross, MH; Kaye, GI; Pawlina W. *Histology. A Text and Atlas*, 4th ed. Philadelphia: Lippincott Williams and Wilkins; 2003.

[4] Căruntu, ID; Cotuţiu, C. *Histologie. Ţesuturi fundamentale*. Iaşi: Ed. Gr. T. Popa; 2004.

[5] Grigoraş, A; Floarea-Strat, A. *Histologie ilustrată*. Iaşi: Ed. Junimea; 2009.

[6] Gartner, LP; Hiatt, JL. *Color Texbook of Histology*, 3th ed. Philadelphia: Saunders; 2007.

[7] Junqueira, LC; Carneiro, J. *Basic Histology: Text and Atlas,* 11th ed. Connecticut: McGraw-Hill/Appleton and Lange; 2005.

[8] Eroschenko, VP. *di Fiore' s Atlas of Histology with Functional Correlations*, 11th ed. Philadelphia: Lippincott Williams and Wilkins; 2007.

[9] Ulmeanu, R; Mihălţan, FD; Cordoş, I; Ulmeanu, DI. *Actualităţi în endoscopia toracică diagnostică şi terapeutică,* Bucureşti: Ed. Universitară Carol Davila; 2009.

[10] Ciobanu, L. *Ghiduri de practică şi protocoale în fibrobronhos*copie. Iaşi: Ed. Fides; 2001.

[11] Van Vyve, V; Chanez, P; Bousquet, J; Lacoste, JY; Michel, FB; Godard, P. Safety of bronchoalveolar lavage and bronchial biopsies in patients with asthma of variable severity. *Am. Rev. Respir. Dis.* 1992; 146:116-121.

[12] Jarjour, NN; Calhoun, WJ. Bronchoalveolar lavage in stable asthmatics does not cause pulmonary inflammation. *Am. Rev. Respir. Dis.* 1990; 142:100-103.

[13] Djukanovic, R; Wilson, JW; Lai, CK; Holgate, ST; Howarth, PH. The safety aspects of fiberoptic bronchoscopy, bronchoalveolar lavage, and endobronchial biopsy in asthma. *Am. Rev. Respir. Dis.* 1991; 143:772–777.

[14] Humbert, M, Robinson DS, Assoufi B, Kay AB, Durham SR. Safety of fiberoptic bronchoscopy in asthmatic and control subjects and effect on asthma control over two weeks. *Thorax,* 1996; 51:664-669.

[15] Workshop summary and guidelines: investigative use of bronchoscopy, lavage, and bronchial biopsies in asthma and other airway diseases. *J. Allergy Clin. Immunol.* 1991; 88(5):808-814.

[16] Elston, WJ; Whittaker, AJ; Khan, LN; Flood-Page, P; Ramsay, C; Jeffery, PK; Barnes, NC. Safety of research bronchoscopy, biopsy and bronchoalveolar lavage in asthma. *Eur. Respir. J.* 2004; 24(3):375-377.

[17] Laitinen, LA; Heino, M; Laitinen, A; Kava, T; Haahtela, T. Damage of the airway epithelium and bronchial reactivity in patients with asthma. *Am. Rev. Respir. Dis.* 1985; 131:599-606.

[18] Jeffery, PK; Wardlaw, AJ; Nelson, FC; Collins, JV; Kay, AB. Bronchial biopsies in asthma: an ultrastructural quantitative study and correlation with hyperreactivity. *Am. Rev. Respir. Dis.* 1989; 140:1745-1753.

[19] Naylor, B. The shedding of the mucosa of the bronchial tree in asthma. *Thorax,* 1962; 17:69-72.

[20] Kirby, JG; Hargreave, FE; Gleich, GJ; O'Byrne, PM. Bronchoalveolar cell profiles of asthmatic and non-asthmatic subjects. *Am. Rev. Respir. Dis.* 1987; 136:379-383.
[21] Ordonez, C; Ferrando, R; Hyde, MD; Wong, HH; Fahy, VJ. Epithelial Desquamation in Asthma Artifact or Pathology? *Am. J. Respir. Crit. Care Med.* 2000; 162(6): 2324-2329.
[22] Fahy, VJ. Remodeling of the airway epithelium in asthma. *Am. J. Respir. Crit. Care Med.* 2001; 164:S46-51.
[23] Fahy, JV; Liu, J; Wong, H; Boushey, HA. Analysis of cellular and biochemical constituents of induced sputum after allergen challenge: a method for studying allergic airway inflammation. *J. Allergy Clin. Immunol.* 1994; 93:1031-1039.
[24] Redington, A; Springall, D; Ghatel, M; Lau, LC; Bloom, S; Holgate, S; Polak, J; Howarth, P. Endothelin in bronchoalveolar lavage fluid and its relation to airflow obstruction in asthma. *Am. J. Respir. Crit. Care Med.* 1995; 151:1034-1039.
[25] Wegner, CD; Rothlein, R; Gundel, RH. Adhesion molecules in the pathogenesis of asthma. *Agents Actions Suppl.* 1991; 34:529-544.
[26] Liu, C; Xiang, Y; Liu, H; Li, Y; Tan, Y; Zhu, X; Zeng, D; Li, M; Zhang, L; Qin X. Integrin beta4 was downregulated on the airway epithelia of asthma patients. *Acta Biochim. Biophys. Sin. (Shanghai)* 2010; 42(8):538-547.
[27] Holgate, ST. The airway epithelium is central to the pathogenesis of asthma. *Allergol. Int.* 2008; 57(1):1-10.
[28] Holgate, ST. Epithelium dysfunction in asthma. *J. Allergy Clin. Immunol.* 2007; 120(6):1233-1244.
[29] Guyton, AC. *Tratat de fiziologie a omului*, 11th ed. București: Ed. Medicală Calisto; 2007.
[30] Patton, KT; Thibodeau, GA; Douglas, MM. *Essentials of Anatomy and Physiology*. Amsterdam: Elsevier; 2011.
[31] Sumi, Y; Hamid, Q. Airway remodeling in asthma. *Allergol. Int.* 2007; 56(4):341-348.
[32] Fahy, JV. Goblet cell and mucin gene abnormalities in asthma. *Chest,* 2002; 122(6):320-326.
[33] Rogers, DF. The airway goblet cell. *Int. J. Biochem. Cell Biol.* 2003; 35(1):1-6.
[34] Rogers, DF. Airway goblet cells: responsive and adaptable front-line defenders. *Eur. Respir. J.* 1994; 7(9):1690-1706.

[35] Groneberg, DA; Eynott, PR; Lim, S; Oates, T; Wu, R; Carlstedt, I; Roberts, P; McCann, B; Nicholson, AG; Harrison, BD; Chung, KF. Expression of respiratory mucins in fatal status asthmaticus and mild asthma. *Histopathology,* 2002; 40(4):367-373.

[36] Ordoñez, C; Khashayar, R; Wong, H; Ferrando, R; Wu, R; Hyde, DM; Hotchkiss, JA; Zhang, Y; Novikov, A; Dolganov, G; Fahy, JV. Mild and moderate asthma is associated with airway goblet cell hyperplasia and abnormalities in mucin gene expression. *Am. J. Respir. Crit. Care Med.* 2001; 163(2):517-523.

[37] Morcillo, EJ; Cortijo, J. Mucus and MUC in asthma. *Curr. Opin. Pulm. Med.* 2006; 12(1):1-6.

[38] Rose, MC; Voynow, JA. Respiratory tract mucin genes and mucin glycoproteins in health and disease. *Physiol. Rev.* 2006; 86(1):245–278.

[39] Hovenberg, HW; Davies, JR; Herrmann, A; Linden, CJ; Carlstedt, I. MUC5AC, but not MUC2, is a prominent mucin in respiratory secretions. *Glycoconj J.* 1996; 13(5):839–847.

[40] Davies, JR; Herrmann, A; Russell, W; Svitacheva, N; Wickstrom, C; Carlstedt, I. Respiratory tract mucins: structure and expression patterns. *Novartis Found Symp.* 2002; 248:76–88.

[41] Rubin, BK. Physiology of airway mucus clearance. *Respir. Care,* 2002; 47(7):761-768.

[42] Thornton, DJ; Howard, M; Khan, N; Sheehan, JK. Identification of two glycoforms of the MUC5B mucin in human respiratory mucus. Evidence for a cysteine-rich sequence repeated within the molecule. *J. Biol. Chem.* 1997; 272(14):9561–9566.

[43] Sheehan, JK; Richardson, PS; Fung, DC; Howard, M; Thornton, DJ. Analysis of respiratory mucus glycoproteins in asthma: a detailed study from a patient who died in status asthmaticus. *Am. J. Respir. Cell Mol. Biol.* 1995; 13(6):748–756.

[44] Rogers, DF; Barnes, PJ. Treatment of airway mucus hypersecretion. *Ann. Med.* 2006; 38(2):116-125.

[45] Xiang, J; Rir-Sim-Ah, J; Tesfaigzi, Y. IL-9 and IL-13 induce mucous metaplasia that is reduced by IFN-gamma in a Bax-mediated pathway. *Am. J. Respir. Cell Mol. Biol.* 2008; 38(3):310-317.

[46] Ricciardolo, F; Di Stefano, A; van Krieken, J; Sont, J; van Schadewijk, A; Rabe, K; Donner, C; Hiemstra, P; Sterk, P; Mauad, T. Proliferation and inflammation in bronchial epithelium after allergen in atopic asthmatics. *Clin. Exp. Allergy,* 2003; 33:905–911.

[47] Vignola, AM; Chiappara, G; Siene, L; Bruno, A; Gagliardo, R; Merendino, AM; Polla, BS; Arrigo, AP; Bonsignore, G; Bousquet, J; Chanez, P. Proliferation and activation of bronchial epithelial cells in corticosteroid-dependent asthma. *J. Allergy Clin. Immunol.* 2001; 108(5):738-746.
[48] Druilhe, A; Wallaert, B; Tsicopoulos, A; Lapa e Silva, JR; Tillie-Leblond, I; Tonnel, AB; Pretolani, M. Apoptosis, proliferation and expression of Bcl-2, Fas, and Fas Ligand in bronchial biopsies from asthmatics. *Am. J. Respir. Cell Mol. Biol.* 1998; 19(5):747-745.
[49] Cohen, L; Tarsi, J; Ramkumar, T; Horiuchi, TK; Cochran, R; DeMartino, S. Epithelial cell proliferation contributes to airway remodeling in severe asthma. *Am. J. Respir. Crit. Care Med.* 2007; 176(2):138-145.
[50] Grigoraş, CC; Grigoraş, A; Mihăescu, T; Vereş, L; Carasevici, E. Nivelul expresiei factorului de proliferare Ki-67 în astmul bronşic. *Rev. Med. Chir. Soc. Med. Nat. Iaşi.* 2009; 113(4):1034-1039.
[51] Alnemri, ES; Livingston, DJ; Nicholson, DW; Salvesen, G; Thornberry, NA; Wong, WW; Yuan, J. Human ICE/CED-3 protease nomenclature. *Cell,* 1996; 87:171.
[52] Green, DR; Reed, JC. Mitochondria and apoptosis. *Science,* 1998; 281:1309–1312.
[53] Wallach, D; Varfolomeev, EE; Malinin, NL; Goltsev, YV; Kovalenko, AV; Boldin, MP. Tumor necrosis factor receptor and Fas signaling mechanisms. *Annu. Rev. Immunol.* 1999; 17:331–367.
[54] Oltvai, ZN; Milliman, CL; Korsmeyer, SJ. Bcl-2 hetero-dimerizes in vivo with a conserved homolog, Bax, that accelerates programmed cell death. *Cell,* 1993; 74:609–619.
[55] Zalewski, PD; Ruffin, RE. Apoptosis-regulatory factors as potential drug targets in the epithelium of normal and inflamed airways. *Curr. Mol. Pharmacol.* 2008; 1:38-49.
[56] Hackett, TL; Knight, DA. The role of epithelial injury and repair in the origins of asthma. *Curr. Opin. Allergy Clin. Immunol.* 2007; 7:63-68.
[57] Tesfaigzi, Y. Roles of apoptosis in airway epithelia. *Am. J. Respir. Cell Mol. Biol.* 2006; 34: 537-547.
[58] Jyonouchi, H. Airway epithelium and apoptosis. *Apoptosis,* 1999; 4:407-417.
[59] Vignola, MA; Mirabella, F; Costanzo, G; Di Giorgo, R; Gjomarkaj, M; Bellia, V; Bonsignore, G. Airway remodeling in asthma. *Chest,* 2003; 123:417-422.

[60] Grigoras, A; Grigoras, CC; Mihăescu, T; Veres, L; Cotutiu, C; Floarea-Strat, A. Apoptosis quantification at the respiratory epithelium level in asthma. *Cent. Eur. J. Med.* 2010; 5(5):556-564.

[61] Schwalm, K; Stevens, JF; Jiang, Z; Schuyler, MR; Schrader, R; Randell, SH; Green, FH; Tesfaigzi, Y. Expression of the proapoptotic protein Bax is reduced in bronchial mucous cells of asthmatic subjects. *Am. J. Physiol. Lung Cell Mol. Physiol.* 2008; 294(6):1102-1129.

[62] Shi, ZQ; Feng, Y; Hou, YK; Liu, T; Xiu, QY. A study of interferon-gamma induced airway mucous cell apoptosis and its mechanisms. *Zhonghua Jie He He Hu Xi Za Zhi* 2005; 28(3):160-163.

[63] Xiang, J; Rir-Sim-Ah, J; Tesfaigzi, Y. IL-9 and IL-13 induce mucous cell metaplasia that is reduced by IFN-gamma in a Bax-mediated pathway. *Am. J. Respir. Cell Mol. Biol.* 2008; 38(3):310-7.

[64] Fahy, JV; Corry, DB; Boushey, HA. Airway inflammation and remodeling in asthma. *Curr. Opin. Pulm. Med.* 2000; 6(1):15-20.

[65] Dorscheid, D; Wojcik, K; Sun, S; Marroquin, B; Steven, R. Apoptosis of Airway Epithelial Cells Induced by Corticosteroids. *Am. J. Respir. Crit. Care Med.* 2001; 164(10):1939-1947.

[66] White, S; Delbert, R; Dorscheid, M. Corticosteroid-Induced Apoptosis of Airway Epithelium A Potential Mechanism for Chronic Airway Epithelial Damage in Asthma. *Chest* 2002; 122:278-284.

[67] Esmailpour, N; Högger, P; Rabe, K; Heitmann, U; Nakashima, M; Rohdewald, P. Distribution of inhaled fluticasone propionate between human lung tissue and serum in vivo. *Eur. Respir. J.* 1997; 10:1496-1499.

[68] Truong-Tran, AQ; Grosser, D; Ruffin, RE; Murgia, C; Zalewski, PD. Apoptosis in the normal and inflamed airway epithelium: role of zinc in epithelial protection and procaspase-3 regulation. *Biochem. Pharmacol.* 2003; 66:1459-1468.

[69] Zalewski, PD. Zinc metabolism in the airway: basic mechanisms and drug targets. *Curr. Opin. Pharmacol.* 2006; 6:237-243.

[70] Bao, S; Knoell, DL. Zinc modulates airway epithelium susceptibility to death receptor-mediated apoptosis. *Am. J. Physiol. Lung Cell Mol. Physiol.* 2006; 290:L433-L441.

[71] Maddika, S; Ande, SR; Panigrahi, S; Paranjothy, T; Weglarczyk, K; Zuse, A; Eshraghi, M; Manda, KD; Wiechec, E; Los, M. Cell survival, cell death and cell cycle pathways are interconnected: implications for cancer therapy. *Drug Resist. Updat.* 2007; 10:13-29.

[72] Blundell, R; Harrison, DJ; O'Dea, S. p21(Wafl/Cip1) regulates proliferation and apoptosis in airway epithelial cells and alternative forms have altered binding activities. *Exp. Lung Res.* 2004; 30:447-464.

[73] Fedorov, IA; Wilson, SJ; Davies, ED; Holgate, ST. Epithelial stress and structural remodelling in childhood asthma. *Thorax* 2005; 60:389-394.

[74] Puddicombe, SM; Torres-Lozano, C; Richter, A; Bucchieri, F; Lordan, JL; Howarth, PH; Vrugt, B; Albers, R; Djukanovic, R; Holgate, ST; Wilson, SJ; Davies, DE. Increased expression of p21(waf) cyclin-dependent kinase inhibitor in asthmatic bronchial epithelium. *Am. J. Respir. Cell Mol. Biol.* 2003; 28: 61-68.

[75] Serikov, VB; Leutenegger, C; Krutilina, R; Kropotov, A; Pleskach, N; Suh, JH; Tomilin, NV. Cigarette smoke extract inhibits expression of peroxiredoxin V and increases airway epithelial permeability. *Inhal. Toxicol.* 2006; 18:79-92.

[76] Gelbman, BD; Heguy, A; O'Connor, TP; Zabner, J; Crystal, RG. Up-regulation of pirin expression by chronic cigarette smoking is associated with bronchial epithelial cell apoptosis. *Respir. Res.* 2007; 8:10.

In: Asthma: Causes, Complications and Treatment ISBN: 978-1-62257-447-6
Editors: A. H. Bislimi and L. C. Tolka

Chapter V

Epidemiology of Asthma during Pregnancy

Ohad Katz [*] ***and Eyal Sheiner***
Department of Obstetrics and Gynecology, Soroka University Medical Center, Faculty of Health Sciences, Ben-Gurion University of the Negev, Beer-Sheva, Israel

Introduction

Chronic bronchial asthma is the most commonly encountered respiratory disorder complicating pregnancy and is a potentially serious medical condition that represents a significant public health issue [1–5].

The prevalence of asthma in pregnant women ranges between 0.4% and 12% [1–11] (with an average of 4–8%) and appears to have increased over recent decades. Kwon et al. [7] demonstrated a two-fold increase in the prevalence of asthma from 2.9% to 5.8% between 1976–1980 and 1988–1994. This diversity of statistics is presumably the result of differences in the definitions of asthma [5].

[*] Corresponding author: Ohad Katz, M.D., Department of Obstetrics and Gynecology, Soroka University Medical Center, P.O. Box 151, Beer Sheva 84101, Israel. Tel.: +972-8-640-3762; Fax: +972-8-640-3057; E-mail: katzoh@bgu.ac.il.

Diagnosis and Classification of Severity

Bronchial asthma is a chronic inflammatory airway disorder that is characterized by paroxysmal or persistent symptoms such as wheezing, coughing, sputum production, shortness of breath, or chest tightness. The diagnosis is based on a combination of a history of such symptoms, objective tests of lung function (i.e., an airflow obstruction that is at least partially reversible), and exclusion of alternative diagnoses [12–15].

During pregnancy, as well as in non-pregnant women with asthma, sequential measurement of forced expiratory volume in one second (FEV1) is the single best measure reflecting the severity of the disease. Peak expiratory flow rate (PEFR) is the largest expiratory flow achieved with a maximally forced effort from a position of maximal inspiration. It is usually attained within the initial 1 second of forced expiration. PEFR correlates well with FEV1 and can be measured reliably. Asthmatic patients will demonstrate an improvement in FEV1/PEFR values following administration of bronchodilators such as β2-agonists [12,13].

In 2004, the National Asthma Education and Prevention Program (NAEPP) Working Group on Asthma and Pregnancy classified asthma severity into four categories—mild intermittent, mild persistent, moderate persistent, and severe persistent. This classification was based on two criteria: clinical symptoms and objective pulmonary function tests (PEFR and FEV1). Regular medical treatment was not included as a criterion [12,15].

Physiologic Changes during Pregnancy

Pulmonary system—Throughout pregnancy, the enlarging uterus elevates the diaphragm about 4 cm and increases the transverse diameter of the thoracic cage about 2 cm [12,13]. The sub-costal angle widens appreciably and the thoracic circumference increases about 6 cm [13]. As a consequence, there is a reduction of the functional residual capacity (FRC) and residual volume (RV). Nevertheless, the vital capacity, PEFR, and FEV1 are not altered appreciably [12,13]. These changes result in hyperventilation in 60–70% of normal pregnancies and, occasionally, a sensation of dyspnea [13,14].

Brancazio et al. [16] measured PEFR in 57 women during each trimester and postpartum. PEFRs were normalized according to the accepted standard nomograms. No significant changes were demonstrated during the three trimesters and postpartum. Hassan et al. [17], however, studied the effect of gestational age on PEFR. They measured PEFRs in the standing, sitting, and supine positions in 38 healthy pregnant women at 4-week intervals starting at less than 10 weeks until delivery and again at 6 weeks postpartum. A small but significant decline in PEFR was demonstrated throughout pregnancy with a mean decline rate of 0.65 L/min per week (normal range of PEFR for reproductive women has been reported to be approximately 380–500 L/min). They concluded that PEFR measurements are affected by maternal position and advancing gestational age, especially in the supine position, and recommended an adjustment of patient's flow rate in relation to gestational age and maternal position, especially in pregnant women with asthma.

Gastrointestinal system—approximately one-third of the women have a gastroesophageal reflex disease (GERD) during pregnancy, especially during the second and third trimesters [13,14]. A reflux of gastric content can cause exacerbation of asthma.

Effects of Pregnancy on Asthma

The course of asthma during pregnancy is variable and may be influenced by the various physiologic changes during pregnancy as well as the severity of the pre-existing disease [14]. For many years, based on several historical cohort and prospective studies, the consensus has remained that about one-third of asthmatic women experience worsening of the disease during pregnancy, another third experience some kind of symptomatic improvement, and the rest have no change [3, 5,13,18,19] Nevertheless, it is unclear whether this pattern is due to changes in asthma control, changes in asthma severity, or exacerbations related to pregnancy. Several studies have been done to answer these questions, but most are limited by their subjective nature. Only relatively few of these studies have examined objective measures such as spirometry [5].

The Course of Asthma during Pregnancy

In a multi-center, prospective, observational cohort study, Schatz et al. evaluated the relationship between asthma severity during pregnancy and gestational asthma exacerbations in 1734 asthmatic women. They found that about 30% of the women who were classified as having a mild disease at the beginning of their pregnancy became worse during pregnancy, and 23% of the women who were classified as having a moderate to severe disease improved [20]. In another prospective study, Schatz et al. followed the progression of asthma during pregnancy and puerperium in 330 women. The women were asked to subjectively rate their asthma symptoms during this period of time. Interestingly, 8% of the women who reported an improvement in their disease and 17% of the women who felt no change in their disease had an emergency department presentation for asthma during pregnancy, suggesting that even women who report an improvement in their asthma may require medical intervention during pregnancy [21]. Recently, Murphy et al. reviewed the literature for publications related to asthma exacerbations during pregnancy and found that exacerbations that required medical treatment occurred in about 20% of women [18]. In a prospective cohort study of 146 women, Murphy et al. [18] evaluated asthma exacerbations during pregnancy and observed that the exacerbation rate increased significantly with increasing asthma severity. Only 8% of women with mild asthma experienced an exacerbation compared with 47% of women with moderate asthma and 65% of women with severe asthma at a mean gestational age of 25 weeks. Respiratory viral infections were the most common precipitants of exacerbations (34%), followed by non-adherence to inhaled corticosteroid medication (29%). Exacerbation during labor and delivery were less common – ten to twenty percent [22]. Other investigators reported similar results [23–25]. Stenius-Aarniala et al. investigated, prospectively, 198 asthmatic women during pregnancy; 42% of the women needed more medication, while 18% needed less medication and 40% were managed with the same anti-asthmatic medication as before pregnancy [23].

The findings of these studies challenge the concept mentioned above that only one-third of asthmatic women experience worsening of the disease during pregnancy, and suggest that the real risk of having an exacerbation during pregnancy is underestimated. These results also emphasize the importance of monitoring asthmatic women with pulmonary function testing during pregnancy, regardless of their asthma severity at the beginning of the pregnancy.

Fetal Sex

Several studies examined the possible influences of fetal sex on maternal asthma. In 1998, Beecroft et al. reported a possible association between asthma severity and fetal sex, based on the analysis of a questionnaire by 18 asthmatic women carrying a male fetus and 16 asthmatic women carrying a female fetus. They demonstrated that significantly more pregnant women carrying a female fetus experienced a worsening of symptoms, while pregnant women carrying a male fetus were more likely to report an improvement. The limitation of this study, however, is its small population [26]. One year later, Dodds et al. [27] reported a re-analysis of their population-based study from Canada that supported the association noted by Beecroft et al. Compared with women carrying a female fetus, fewer asthmatic women carrying a male fetus required steroid treatment (20% vs. 14%). Furthermore, more pregnant women carrying a male fetus used β2-agonists alone compared with women carrying a female fetus (40% vs. 35%), suggesting that asthma in pregnant women with a male fetus can be managed better than in pregnant women carrying a female fetus [27]. Between 1997 and 2000, Kwon et al. investigated prospectively the association between fetal sex and maternal airway lability among more than 700 pregnant asthmatic women. They significantly demonstrated a 10% improvement in airway lability among women carrying a male fetus compared with women carrying a female fetus. This difference persisted throughout pregnancy. In the authors' opinion, the assumption that sex hormones modulate asthma severity during pregnancy is reasonable [28]. Recently, Bakhireva et al. prospectively tested this hypothesis using a sample of 719 pregnant women with asthma. Pregnancy with a female fetus was associated with a higher incidence of asthma exacerbations (OR 1.84; 95% CI) independent of maternal age, BMI, ethnicity, smoking, and socioeconomic status [29]. Firoozi et al., however, failed to demonstrate such an association. In a large cohort study they compared 5529 pregnancies with a single female fetus and 5728 pregnancies with a single male fetus that gave birth between 1990 and 2002 in Quebec. No significant differences were found between mothers of a female or male fetus as to the occurrence of asthma exacerbations, the daily dose of inhaled corticosteroides (ICS), and the weekly dose of inhaled short-acting beta agonists (SABA) [30]. Other studies have failed to demonstrate such an association as well [31,32].

There is evidence that by potentiating the β-adrenergic-mediated relaxation of bronchial tissue and inhibiting the response to histamine, testosterone has a protective effect on asthmatic women, particularly from the second trimester onward. Another possible mechanism involves the activation of inflammatory pathways associated with asthma by sex-specific factors related to the female fetus [28]. Nevertheless, the fetal-sex related mechanisms responsible for the changes in the course of asthma during pregnancy are yet to be determined. The available literature has offered conflicting evidence and thus further research with large sample sizes is needed to clarify these potential effects.

Effects of Asthma on Pregnancy

A review of the studies investigating the association between maternal asthma and adverse pregnancy and perinatal outcomes reveals inconsistent data. While several studies have found an association between asthma and increased risk for adverse maternal and perinatal outcomes, other studies have failed to demonstrate such an association, especially among women with a better controlled disease (i.e., reduced number of exacerbations or higher maternal pulmonary function) [1,3,4].

Table 1. Effects of maternal asthma on pregnancy outcomes—retrospective studies

Author [Year] ref.	Country	Control	Asthma	Significant association to asthma	No association to asthma
Lao and Huensgsburg (1990) [17]	Hong Kong	87	87	Low birth weight, Cesarean delivery	
Perlow et al. (1992) [38]	US	130	81	Cesarean delivery, preterm labor, low birth weight	Pre-eclampsia, IUGR, congenital malformations
Lehrer et al. (1993) [39]	US	22,680	1571	Pregnancy induced hypertension	
Demissie et al. (1998) [40]	US	9156	2289	Low birth weight, preterm delivery, pre-eclampsia, congenital malformations, cesarean delivery	
Alexander et al. (1998) [6]	Canada	13709	817	Ante/postpartum hemorrhage, pregnancy induced hypertension (with steroid treatment)	Preterm delivery, pregnancy induced hypertension, Cesarean delivery
Kallen et al. (2000) [35]	Sweden	1.32M	36985	Preterm and postterm delivery, perinatal mortality, Low birth weight	Congenital malformations

Author [Year] ref.	Country	Control	Asthma	Significant association to asthma	No association to asthma
Wen et al. (2001) [42]	Canada	34,668	8672	Pre-eclampsia, preterm delivery, low birth weight	Fetal death
Liu et al. (2001) [41]	Canada	8772	2193	Pre-eclampsia, preterm delivery, small for gestational age, Cesarean delivery	Congenital malformations
Norjavaara and de Verdier (2003) [43]	Sweden	293,948	2968	Cesarean delivery	Still birth, Low birth weight, congenital malformations
Sheiner et al. (2005) [4]	Israel	137,205	1963	Cesarean delivery, IUGR	Perinatal mortality, low birth weight
Getahun et al. (2006) [37]	US	36.9M	332,357	Placental abruption - modest (blacks)	
Enriquez et al. (2007) [37]	US	131145	9154	Hypertensive disorders of pregnancy, membrane-related disorders, antepartum hemorrhage, cesarean delivery	Preterm birth, birth defects
Tata et al. (2007) [34]	GBR	24,3434	37,585	Miscarriage, antepartum and postpartum hemorrhage, cesarean delivery	Placental abruption, placenta previa, preeclampsia, hypertension, gestational diabetes, assisted delivery
Katz et al. (2007) [44]	Israel	196,707	2669	Preterm delivery (in winter season)	
Blais and Forget (2008) [36]	Canada		4344	Congenital malformations	
Tata et al. (2008) [45]	GBR			Congenital malformations (OR 1.1)	

Adapted from Katz and Sheiner, Asthma and pregnancy: A review of two decades. Expert Review Respiratory Medicine 2008;2:1-10; with permission of Expert Reviews Ltd.

Table 2. Effects of maternal asthma on pregnancy outcomes—prospective studies

Author [Year] ref.	Country	Control	Asthma	Significant association to asthma	No association to asthma
Stenius-Aarniala et al. (1988) [23]	Finland	198	181	Pre-eclampsia (severe > mild), Cesarean delivery	Low birth weight, preterm delivery, perinatal mortality, congenital malformations
Doucette and Bracken (1993) [51]	US	3859	32	Preterm delivery	Low birth weight
Jana et al. (1995) [25]	India	364	182	Low birth weight (in 15 women who had exacerbations)	Preterm delivery, low birth weight, perinatal mortality
Schatz et al. (1995) [8]	US	486	486		Preterm delivery, perinatal mortality, low birth weight, pre-eclampsia, congenital malformations
Stenius-Aarniala et al. (1996) [49]	Finland	237	504	Cesarean delivery	Preterm delivery, perinatal mortality
Minerbi-Codish et al. (1998) [52]	Israel	77	101		Low birth weight, gestational hypertension, preterm delivery
Sobande et al. (2002) [54]	Saudi Arabia	10	88	Pre-eclampsia, Cesarean delivery, perinatal mortality, low birth weight	
Mihrshahi et al. (2003) [53]	Australia	271	340	hypertension	Cesarean delivery, pre-eclampsia, low birth weight
Bracken et al. (2003) [46]	US	1333	872	Reduction of gestational age at delivery (with oral steroids or theophyline), intrauterine growth restriction	Preterm delivery

Author [Year] ref.	Country	Control	Asthma	Significant association to asthma	No association to asthma
Triche et al. (2004) [47]	US	1052	656	Pre-eclampsia (with moderate and severe asthma)	
Dombrowski et al. (2004) [48]	US	881	1739	Cesarean delivery (with moderate or severe asthma), preterm delivery < 37 weeks (with severe asthma)	Preterm delivery < 32 or 37 weeks, pre-eclampsia
Murphy et al. (2005) [22]	Australia		146	Low birth weight in males (in 53 women who had exacerbations)	
Bakhireva et al. (2008) [50]	US		716	Preterm delivery	IUGR

Adapted from Katz and Sheiner, Asthma and pregnancy: A review of two decades. Expert Review Respiratory Medicine 2008;2:1-10; with permission of Expert Reviews Ltd.

The major retrospective and prospective studies investigating the association between maternal asthma and pregnancy/perinatal outcomes in the past two decades are summarized in Tables 1 and 2.

Retrospective Studies

Recently, Enriquez et al. reported the findings of one of the largest US cohort studies to date, regarding the relationship between maternal asthma, exacerbated asthma, and pregnancy outcomes. After controlling for confounding factors, there were dose-dependent relationships between asthma alone and exacerbated asthma with hypertensive disorders of pregnancy, membrane-related disorders, preterm labor, antepartum hemorrhage, and cesarean delivery. Maternal asthma was not associated with preterm birth or birth defects. They concluded that asthma is a risk factor for several common adverse outcomes of pregnancy, and poorly controlled asthma during pregnancy increases these risks [33].

The same year, Tata et al. [34] reported the results of a comprehensive analysis of adverse obstetric outcomes in women with and without asthma. All codes relating to stillbirth, miscarriage, therapeutic abortion, and obstetric complications were extracted from the Health Improvement Network database for (281,019) pregnancies between 1988 and 2004. Data regarding socioeconomic status and behavioral characteristics were extracted as well. Asthma severity was categorized into three levels according to the British Thoracic Society asthma guidelines for medication use. The unit of analysis was a pregnancy. Odds ratios of the outcomes comparing pregnancies in women with and without asthma were estimated using a logistic regression analysis. In 37,585 pregnancies of asthmatic women the risk of miscarriage was slightly higher (OR 1.10; 95% CI 1.06–1.13) than that of non-asthmatic women. The risks of stillbirth and therapeutic abortion, however, were similar. Risks of most obstetric complications (placental abruption, placenta previa, preeclampsia, hypertension, gestational diabetes, and assisted delivery) were not higher among asthmatic women, with the exception of increases in antepartum (OR 1.20; 95% CI 1.08–1.34) or postpartum (OR 1.38; 95% CI 1.21–1.57) hemorrhage, and caesarean section (OR 1.11; 95% CI 1.07–1.16). Risks of miscarriage and caesarean section increased moderately in women with more severe asthma and previous asthma exacerbations. According to the authors, these results indicate that asthmatic women have similar reproductive risks compared with women without asthma in the general population for most of the range of outcomes studied.

A few years earlier, Källén et al. [35] published the results of one of the largest retrospective studies on pregnancy outcomes in asthmatic women to date. They analyzed the pregnancy outcomes of nearly 37,000 asthmatic women who gave birth between 1984 and 1985. The analysis results were compared with the total births that occurred in Sweden during the same period of time (more than 1.3 million). Contrary to Tata et al., they found that the pregnancies of asthmatic women were significantly more likely to be complicated by preterm delivery, prolonged pregnancy (more than 41 weeks), low birth weight, pre-eclampsia, and perinatal mortality, with a correlation to asthma severity. No association to congenital malformations was noted.

Blais and Forget [36] conducted a large retrospective study of 4344 pregnancies of asthmatic women to investigate the association between first trimester exacerbations and increased risk for congenital malformations. The crude prevalence of malformations was 12.8% for women who had an exacerbation during the first trimester and 8.9% for women who did not. A 50% increased risk of congenital malformations was demonstrated for women who had an asthma exacerbation during the first trimester of pregnancy. Although it has limitations (residual confounding might be present and part of the observed association might be due to the use of oral corticosteroids), this study adds evidence to the necessity of keeping asthma under control during pregnancy to avoid exacerbations.

Getahun et al. [37] investigated the associations between maternal respiratory diseases and abruption in the United States. Data on women who delivered singleton births (n = 37,314,022) were derived from the National Hospital Discharge Survey for 1993 to 2003. ICD-9-CM codes were used to identify pregnant women hospitalized for respiratory disease and for placental abruption. RR and 95% CI were derived from multivariable logistic regression models to evaluate the associations after adjusting for maternal sociodemographic and behavioral characteristics. The association between asthma and abruption was modest (RR 1.1, 95% CI 1.0–1.2). Stratified analysis by maternal race showed that asthma was associated with abruption among black women but not white women.

The variable pregnancy outcomes were demonstrated by earlier studies as well. Lao and Huengsburg investigated pregnancy outcomes of 87 asthmatic women in Hong Kong between 1984 and 1987. Pregnancies of asthmatic women were significantly more likely to be complicated by preterm delivery (especially those who did not use medications) or cesarean delivery [19].

Perlow et al. [38] demonstrated an increased risk for preterm delivery and cesarean delivery, and low birth weight among women with severe asthma (oral steroid dependent). No association with pre-eclampsia or congenital malformations was noted. Nevertheless, this study included 187 asthmatic women and has a low power to detect such effects.

In a large study of about 24,000 women, of whom nearly 1,600 were asthmatic, Lehrer et al. [39] found a significant association between pregnancy-induced hypertension and asthma. This association persisted after adjustment for confounding factors. They also found a significant association between pregnancy-induced hypertension and a history of asthma. Nevertheless, after adjustment for potential confounders, this association failed to achieve statistical significance.

Demissie et al. [40] examined the association between asthma and maternal/perinatal outcomes, using a historical cohort analysis of singleton live deliveries in New Jersey hospitals between 1989 and 1992. A comparison of 2,289 women with an ICD-9-CM diagnosis code for asthma was conducted with a randomly-selected control sample of 9,156 women. After controlling for potential confounders, maternal asthma was significantly associated with preterm delivery, low birth weight, pre-eclampsia, and cesarean delivery. Unlike the previous studies, an increased risk for congenital malformations was noted.

Alexander et al. [6] conducted a similar study in Canada, but unlike the previous studies, during the examination of the medical records, the asthmatic women were classified into three groups of severity based on medication usage (no medication, beta agonist only, steroids). A total of 817 asthmatic women were compared with 13,709 non-asthmatic women for maternal complication and neonatal outcomes. Regardless of medication use, asthma was associated with ante-partum and post-partum hemorrhage. Asthmatic women using steroids were found to be at a slightly increased risk for gestational hypertension, possibly a complication of steroid use [6].

Using the Quebec hospital discharge records for 1991–1992 and 1995–1996, Liu et al. [41] investigated 2,193 asthmatic and 8,772 normal singleton pregnancies. After adjusting for potential confounders, maternal asthma was significantly associated with preterm birth, infants who are very small for gestational age, pre-eclampsia (and transient hypertension of pregnancy), and cesarean delivery. There was no association to congenital malformations. Wen et al. [42] demonstrated similar results.

Norjavaara et al. [43] investigated the influences of inhaled steroids on pregnancy outcomes during 1995 to 1998. Nearly 3,000 asthmatic women who used inhaled budesonide were compared to 7,700 women who used other asthma medications and to a control group of more than 293,000 healthy women. Other than cesarean delivery, the use of inhaled budesonide was not linked with any adverse pregnancy outcome.

Sheiner et al. [4] conducted a large retrospective population-based study, investigating pregnancy outcomes among asthmatic women. They compared all singleton pregnancies of asthmatic (1,963) and non-asthmatic (137,205) mothers who delivered between 1988 and 2002 in the Soroka University Medical Center (the sole hospital in the Negev, the southern part of Israel, which serves the entire obstetrical population in this region). After adjusting for potential confounders, the following adverse outcomes were associated with asthma: intrauterine growth restriction, hypertensive disorders, premature rapture of membranes, and cesarean delivery. Nevertheless, perinatal outcome was favorable.

Our group had investigated the seasonal effect on singleton deliveries, comparing all singleton pregnancies of asthmatic (n=2669) and non-asthmatic (n=196,707) women who gave birth between 1988 and 2006 [44]. A higher rate of preterm delivery was noted during the winter season among patients residing in semi-nomadic settlements compared to sedentary cities. Recently, Tata et al. [45] evaluated the association of maternal asthma and exposure to asthma medications during pregnancy with the risk of major congenital malformations. The unit of analysis was the child. A conditional logistic regression was used to assess the association of any major congenital malformation with maternal asthma and maternal asthma treatment. Live-born children with major congenital malformations numbering 5,124 cases were matched to 30,053 controls. Risk of any malformation in children born to asthmatic women was slightly higher (adjusted OR 1.10, 95% CI 1.01–1.20). No association, however, was demonstrated in children born to mothers receiving asthma treatment in the year before or during pregnancy. No increased risk of malformation was found with gestational exposures to short- or long-acting beta-agonists, inhaled corticosteroids, oral corticosteroids, or other bronchodilators. They concluded that commonly used asthma medications were found to be safe for use during pregnancy.

Prospective Studies

Large multi-center prospective cohort studies investigated pregnancy outcomes of asthmatic women [46–48]. These studies were unique in that they contained information regarding asthma severity and treatment. Bracken et al. [46] recruited 832 asthmatic women and 1,266 non-asthmatic women as a control group. Symptoms and treatment during pregnancy were closely monitored and recorded, and the women were classified according to the Global Initiative for Asthma guidelines as having mild intermittent, mild persistent, moderate persistent, or severe persistent asthma. Adjusted ORs for the associations between asthma status and pregnancy outcomes (preterm delivery and IUGR) were calculated from multiple logistic regression models. Preterm delivery was not associated with asthma diagnosis, regardless of severity classification. However, the need for treatment with daily oral steroid or theophylline was associated with reduction of gestational age at delivery by 2 weeks and 1 week, respectively. An increased risk IUGR was associated with severity of daily symptoms but not with medication type. In another analysis of the same prospective cohort study, Triche and Bracken [47] found that moderate to severe asthma symptoms are significantly associated with an increased risk for pre-eclampsia, regardless of asthma diagnosis or treatment before pregnancy. These results suggest that poor asthma control may affect maternal and fetal outcomes, possibly as a result of chronic maternal hypoxia and/or progressive inflammatory process.

Dombrowski et al. [48] conducted a multi-center prospective observational cohort study involving 16 university hospital centers. Preterm delivery of less than 32 weeks was the primary outcome; secondary outcome measures included pregnancy and neonatal outcomes. Asthma severity was defined according to the NAEPP classification and modified to include medication requirements. A total of 2,620 women were enrolled, of whom 873 had mild asthma, 814 had moderate asthma, and 52 had severe asthma; 881 non-asthmatic women served as a control group. In contrast to the study of Bracken et al., most of the asthmatic women were actively managed, including lung function testing. No significant differences in the rates of preterm delivery of less than 32 or 37 weeks of gestation were noted. Of all the other pregnancy outcomes explored, there were no significant differences for maternal complications except for an increase in overall cesarean delivery rate among the moderate/severe group compared with controls. After adjustment for confounding variables, however, preterm delivery less than 37 weeks and gestational diabetes were associated with severe asthma, most probably due to oral steroid use. These results, with regard to gestation age at delivery and oral steroid use, are similar to those of Bracken et al.

Over a decade earlier, Stenius-Aarniala et al. [49] prospectively followed 198 pregnancies of asthmatic women in Finland. Women were classified as having very mild, mild, moderately severe, or severe asthma. Information regarding the control group was collected retrospectively from labor records of women matched for age, parity, and gestational age. Asthma was significantly associated with mild pre-eclampsia compared with control subjects (15% vs. 5%) and occurred more often among women with severe asthma, compared to women with mild asthma (29% vs. 9%). The use of systemic corticosteroid was also associated with a higher rate of pre-eclampsia [23]. Several years later, the same group prospectively followed 504 pregnant women with asthma. As in their previous study, information regarding the control group was collected retrospectively from labor records of women matched for age, parity, and gestational age. Data on asthmatics with an acute exacerbation during pregnancy were compared with those with no recorded acute exacerbation and with the controls. Women who experienced an acute exacerbation were less likely to have used inhaled corticosteroids (ICS) prior to the exacerbation (17% vs. 4%). With regard to pregnancy outcomes, however, no significant differences were noted between the groups. The prompt use of ICS with these patients may have contributed to the reassuring outcomes [49].

Recently, Bakhireva et al. [50] evaluated the effect of maternal asthma on fetal growth and preterm delivery. A total of 719 pregnant asthmatic women were asked to evaluate their asthma control repeatedly during pregnancy and report hospitalizations and unscheduled clinic visits for asthma exacerbations. Independent of systemic corticosteroid treatment and other covariates, the incidence of preterm delivery was significantly higher among patients with inadequate asthma control during the first part of pregnancy (11.4%) compared with patients with adequate asthma control (6.3%). Similar results were demonstrated among patients who were hospitalized for asthma during pregnancy (16.4%) compared with patients without such history (7.6%). No such association was demonstrated with regard to IUGR. This study demonstrates a substantial risk for preterm delivery posed by poorly controlled maternal asthma and provides additional evidence regarding the importance of adequate treatment of asthma in pregnancy to maintain optimal asthma control.

Review of the recent prospective literature indicates that these results are consistent in the majority of the studies but not in all. Doucette and Bracken [51] compared pregnancy outcomes of 32 asthmatic women to 3,859 controls. Asthma was significantly associated with a two-fold risk for preterm delivery but not with low birth weight. Schatz et al. [8] examined pregnancy outcomes of 486 actively managed asthmatic women and the same number of controls. There were no significant differences between the groups with regard to pre-eclampsia, preterm delivery, IUGR, low birth weight, perinatal mortality, or congenital malformation. Jana et al. [25] reported similar findings in a study of 182 asthmatic and 364 non-asthmatic pregnant women that was conducted in India in 1983–1992. They found no significant increase in adverse pregnancy outcomes among asthmatic women. Nevertheless, in 15 asthmatic women who had a severe exacerbation during the pregnancy, a significant reduction in birth weight was noted. Minerbi-Codish et al. [52] compared 77 asthmatic mothers to 101 controls. Asthmatics were classified as mild, moderate, and severe according to their medical treatment. No significant association was found between maternal asthma or maternal use of corticosteroids and the following outcomes: gestational hypertension, low birth weight, preterm delivery, and Apgar scores. Mihrshahi et al. [53] examined pregnancy outcomes of 340 asthmatic and 271 non-asthmatic women. Asthma was not associated with increased risk for preterm delivery, low birth weight, pre-eclampsia cesarean delivery, and other outcomes. However, a limitation of this study is that women were recruited at 36 weeks' gestation, which may have led to an under-estimation of the adverse effects of asthma on pregnancy outcomes. By contrast, Sobande et al. [54] reported that compared to non-asthmatic women, pregnant asthmatic women are at increased risk for pre-eclampsia, perinatal mortality, low birth weight, and congenital malformations, but not for preterm delivery.

Summary: Effects of Asthma on Pregnancy

In contrast to the newer prospective studies, there is much less consensus among the retrospective studies with regard to pregnancy outcomes. Review of the retrospective literature reveals that asthma has been, but also has *not* been, associated with nearly every possible pregnancy complication. This inconsistency can be partially explained by the fact that the majority of these retrospective studies are limited by the little available information regarding asthma severity or treatment. Furthermore, many of the older studies have several methodologic inadequacies such as low power, lacking control for confounders, different inclusion/exclusion criteria.

The newer prospective studies have the advantage of being able to monitor clinical symptoms or effectiveness of treatment. However, the variation in population characteristics (general treatment, medication type, different criteria for severity classification) makes the comparison between the studies difficult.

Most of the prospective studies published in the past two decades indicate that adverse pregnancy outcomes are infrequent among asthmatic women with a well-controlled disease [8,23,25,52,53]. The two largest studies, by Dombrowski et al. [48] and Bracken et al. [46] (which contained information regarding asthma severity and treatment), indicate that therapy tailored to asthma severity can result in favorable pregnancy outcomes. Severe asthma, however, was found to be associated with an increased risk for preterm delivery, IUGR, and cesarean delivery.

An increased rate of cesarean delivery was also reported by other studies [23,48,50]. A recently published study provides a possible explanation for this finding. Linton and Peterson [55] reported that preexisting chronic conditions, including bronchial asthma, may increase the likelihood that a woman will deliver by cesarean section. It seems that uncertainly in guiding the delivery of asthmatic women, together with the misperception of increased risk of complications, account for the higher rate of cesarean deliveries among those women.

Contrary to previous retrospective publications [6,41,42], the majority of controlled prospective studies found no significant association between well-treated asthma and pre-eclampsia [8,46,48,52,53]. Triche et al. [47], however, found that moderate and severe asthma is significantly associated with an increased risk for pre-eclampsia, regardless of asthma diagnosis or treatment. Schatz [10] suggested that a release of local mediators during an asthma attack can be one of the mechanisms to explain this association. Other suggested mechanisms include hypoxia, inflammation, medication, and smoking [8,37,40-42].

In conclusion, there is extensive evidence that mild or moderate well-controlled asthma can result in excellent pregnancy and perinatal outcomes, whereas severe or poorly controlled asthma may result in adverse maternal and fetal outcomes such as preterm birth, pre-eclampsia, IUGR, and cesarean delivery.

Pharmacologic Therapy

Recently, Belanger et al. [56] concluded that asthma severity during pregnancy is similar to severity during the year before pregnancy, provided patients continued to use their prescribed medication.According to the NAEPP Working Group Report on Managing Asthma During Pregnancy: Recommendations for Pharmacologic Treatment—Update 2004, it is safer for pregnant asthmatics to be medically treated than it is for them to have exacerbations. The stepwise approach, in which the dose, number of medications, and frequency of administration are changed in correlation to asthma severity, is used to achieve and maintain asthma control. For each step medications are defined as "preferred" or "alternative". Patients failing to respond are being stepped up. A step-down approach can be considered once control is sustained for several months [15]. Numerous studies examined the efficacy and safety of anti-asthma drug therapy during pregnancy. As a result, extensive evidence exists regarding the safety of the major drug classes.

Inhaled and Systemic Corticosteriods

Inhaled corticosteroids (ICS) are considered the therapy of choice for treating all levels of persistent asthma during pregnancy [3,12,15]. As mentioned earlier, Stenius-Aarniala et al. [49] demonstrated that women who experienced an acute exacerbation during pregnancy were less likely to have been using ICS prior to the exacerbation. ICS therapy was not associated with adverse pregnancy outcomes. Wendel et al. [57] prospectively studied 84 pregnant women with asthma exacerbations. The women were randomly assigned to receive either intravenous aminophylline and a beta-2 agonist or ICS (methylprednisolone) and a beta-2 agonist. Intravenous aminophylline offered no therapeutic advantages, while ICS reduced the need for subsequent admissions. Using the Swedish Medical Birth Registry, Källén et al. [58] investigated the incidence of congenital malformations among over 2000 infants whose mothers had used inhaled budesonide for asthma in early pregnancy. No significant differences were demonstrated compared to the general population. Norjavaara and de Verdier [43] investigated, retrospectively, whether the reported use of ICS during pregnancy influenced birth outcomes. 2,968 mothers who reported use of ICS during early pregnancy gave birth to infants of normal gestational age, birth weight, with no increased rate of stillbirths. Schatz et al. [59] evaluated the relationship between asthma medication therapy and adverse perinatal outcomes in 2,123 pregnancies. The use of inhaled beta-2 agonists, ICS, or theophylline was not significantly associated with adverse perinatal outcomes. After adjusting for potential confounders, oral corticosteroid use was significantly associated with both preterm delivery at less than 37 weeks' gestation and low birth weight. Dombrowski et al. [60] compared the efficacy of beclomethasone to oral theophylline for the prevention of asthma exacerbation in a prospective, double-blind, double placebo-controlled randomized clinical trial of pregnant women with moderate asthma. No significant differences were demonstrated between the groups with regard to treatment failure, proportion of peak expiratory flow rate less than 80% predicted, or maternal/perinatal outcomes. The theophylline cohort had a significantly higher incidence of treatment discontinuance caused by side effects. Rahimi et al. [61] reported the results of a meta-analysis of all clinical studies that evaluated the pregnancy and perinatal outcomes in women exposed to ICS. ICS therapy was not associated with increased risk for major malformations, preterm delivery, low birth weight, and pregnancy-induced hypertension. Silverman et al. [62] reported similar results. Recently, Breton et al. [63] investigated the effect of ICS use among asthmatic patients on perinatal mortality rate. They compared 4140 asthmatic women who used less than 250 μg/d ICS with 1,140 women who used more than 250 μg/d ICS, and with 7,724 nonusers of ICSs during pregnancy. No significant differences in perinatal mortality were noted between women exposed to ICSs (any dose) vs. non exposed women (OR,

1.07; 95% CI, 0.70-1.61). They concluded that ICS use during pregnancy is not associated with an increased risk for perinatal mortality.

In summary, the consistent findings provided by these studies indicate that ICS therapy is not associated with adverse pregnancy outcomes and is relatively safe for use during pregnancy. The safety of oral steroid treatment during pregnancy, however, is less clear. As mentioned earlier, an association between oral steroid treatment and an increased risk for preterm delivery was demonstrated by the two large prospective cohort studies of Dombrowski et al. [48] and Bracken et al. [46].

Beta-2 Agonists and Theophylline

Inhaled beta-2 agonists are recommended for all degrees of asthma during pregnancy [12] and, according to the NAEPP recommendations [15] (based on a review of six studies), inhaled beta-2 agonists are relatively safe to be used during pregnancy. As noted earlier, Schatz et al. [59] did not find an association between beta-2 agonist use and adverse pregnancy outcomes. Recently, Martel et al. [64] investigated, using a retrospective analysis, the effects of inhaled beta-2 agonists use on the risk of gestational hypertensive disorders (gestational hypertension, pre-eclampsia, eclampsia). Surprisingly, they found that use of inhaled beta-2 agonist during pregnancy was associated with reduced risk. The main effect of thophylline is airway smooth muscle relaxation. The immunomodulatory effects of theophylline are obtained at low plasma concentrations (< 10 mg/L). The combination of ICS and theophylline exerts a synergistic anti-inflammatory effect that improves asthma control and reduces exacerbations [65]. According to the NAEPP recommendations [15] (based upon a review of eight studies) theophylline is relatively safe for use during pregnancy at a serum concentration of 5–12 μg/mL. As noted earlier, the two large prospective studies of Dombrowski et al. and Schatz et al. confirmed these recommendations. Dombrowski's group [48] found that ICS and oral theophylline have the same efficacy in prevention of asthma exacerbation. Nevertheless, the theophylline cohort had a significantly higher incidence of treatment discontinuance caused by side effects. Schatz et al. [59] found that therapy with theophylline as well as with ICS or inhaled beta-2 agonists was not significantly associated with adverse perinatal outcomes.

Combined Therapy

Källén and Otterblad Olausson [66–68] conducted a large retrospective cohort study of over 24,000 pregnant asthmatics who reported the use of anti-asthmatic drugs in early pregnancy. They investigated the association between use of anti-asthmatic drugs during pregnancy and pregnancy complications, the risk for congenital malformations, and perinatal outcomes. The following complications occurred at an increased rate with the use of anti-asthmatic drugs, especially when three or more drugs had been used: preeclampsia, gestational diabetes, hemorrhage, premature rupture of membranes, labor induction, and cesarean delivery. Most of the increased risk for caesarean delivery (OR=1.79) could be explained by these pregnancy complications. Congenital malformations: After adjustment for confounding factors, a weak association between anti-asthmatic drug use and the risk for a congenital malformation was demonstrated (OR=1.09), specifically cardiac defects, orofacial clefts, and anal atresia. The use of inhaled corticosteroids showed a higher odds ratio for orofacial clefts and anal atresia, but the differences could be random. The authors concluded that "The use of anti-asthmatic drugs carry no major risk for congenital malformations, but a slight teratogenic effect cannot be excluded. It may be due to asthma, and arguments for a stronger effect of inhaled corticosteroids than of other anti-asthmatics are weak." Perinatal outcomes: An increased risk for preterm birth (OR=1.46), low birth weight (OR=1.67), small for gestational age (OR=1.70), hyperglycemia (OR=1.62), and mortality (OR=1.52) was found, with correlation to the number of drugs used by the mother during pregnancy, especially when three or more drugs had been used. An increased risk for neonatal icterus was mainly an effect of preterm birth. They concluded that "Infants whose mothers had asthma had a number of manifestations of poor outcome which appeared to be linked with the severity of the asthma."

Conclusion

Asthma is the most common respiratory disorder complicating pregnancy, with an increasing prevalence over recent years. The recent prospective studies investigating the influences of pregnancy on the course of asthma challenge the long-standing consensus that asthma will worsen in one-third, remain unchanged in one-third, and improve in one-third, and suggest that the real risk of having an exacerbation during pregnancy may be underestimated. Despite the controversy between retrospective and prospective cohort studies, it is clear that mild/moderate asthma, managed according to the NAEPP recommendations, is associated with favorable maternal and perinatal outcomes, while severe asthma or untreated asthma may be associated with increased risk for preterm birth, pre-eclampsia, IUGR, and cesarean delivery.

Management of asthma during pregnancy should include objective assessment of lung function, trigger avoidance, patient education, and stepwise therapy. ICS are the preferred treatment for all levels of persistent asthma, but other drug classes are efficient and relatively safe for use as well.

Since asthma is the most common respiratory disorder during pregnancy, further prospective studies should determine its clinical significance during pregnancy, in order to lead to a well-established protocol for surveillance in follow-up during pregnancy.

References

[1] Schatz, M., Zeiger, R. S., Hoffman, C. P. Intrauterine growth is related to gestational pulmonary function in pregnant asthmatic women. Kaiser-Permanente Asthma and Pregnancy Study Group. *Chest* 1990;98:389-92.

[2] Kwon, H. L., Belanger, K., Bracken, M. B. Effect of pregnancy and stage of pregnancy on asthma severity: A systematic review. *Am. J. Obstet. Gynecol.* 2004;190:1201-10.

[3] Namazy, J. A., Schatz, M. Treatment of asthma during pregnancy and perinatal outcomes. *Curr. Opin. Allergy Clin. Immunol.* 2005;5:229-33.

[4] Sheiner, E., Mazor, M., Levy, A., Wiznitzer, A., Bashiri, A. Pregnancy outcome of asthmatic patients: a population-based study. *J. Matern. Fetal. Neonatal Med.* 2005;18:237-40.

[5] Murphy, V. E., Gibson, P. G., Smith, R., Clifton, V. L. Asthma during pregnancy: mechanisms and treatment implications. *Eur. Respir. J.* 2005;25:731-50.

[6] Alexander, S., Dodds, L., Armson, B. A. Perinatal outcomes in women with asthma during pregnancy. *Obstet. Gynecol.* 1998;92:435-40.

[7] Kwon, H. L., Belanger, K., Bracken, M. Asthma prevalence among pregnant and childbearing-aged women in the United States: estimates from national health surveys. *Ann. Epidemiol.* 2003;13:317-24.

[8] Schatz, M., Zeiger, R. S., Hoffman, G. P., Harden, K., Forsythe, A., Chilingar, L., Saunders, B., Porreco, R., Sperling, W., Kagnoff, M., et al.

Perinatal outcomes in the pregnancies of asthmatic women: A prospective controlled analysis. *Am. J. Respir. Crit. Care Med.* 1995;151:1170-4.

[9] Clark, S. L. Asthma in pregnancy. National Asthma Education Program Working Group on Asthma and Pregnancy. National Institutes of Health, National Heart, Lung and Blood Institute. *Obstet. Gynecol.* 1993;82:1036-40.

[10] Schatz, M. Asthma during pregnancy: interrelationships and management. *Ann. Allergy.* 1992;68:123-33.

[11] Katz, O., Sheiner, E. Asthma and pregnancy: A review of two decades. *Expert Rev. Resp. Med.* 2008;2:1-10.

[12] Dombrowski, M. P. Asthma and pregnancy. *Obstet. Gynecol.* 2006;108:667-81.

[13] Cunningham, F. G., Leveno, K. J., Bloom, S. L., Hauth, J. C., Gilstrap, L. C., Wenstrom, K. D., eds. *Williams Obstetrics*, 22nd ed. New York: McGraw-Hill Medical Publishing Division; 2006:136.

[14] Gluck, J. C. The change of asthma course during pregnancy. *Clin. Rev. Allergy Immunol.* 2004;26:171-80.

[15] NAEPP Expert Panel Report. Working Group Report on Managing Asthma During Pregnancy: Recommendations for Pharmacologic Treatment – update 2004. *Allergy Clin. Immunol.* 2005;115:34-46.

[16] Brancazio, L. R., Laifer, S. A., Schwartz, T. Peak expiratory flow rate in normal pregnancy. *Obstet. Gynecol.* 1997;89:383-6.

[17] Hassan, M., Donia, S. E., Nasrallah, F. K., Saade, G. R., Belfort, M. A. Effect of Gestational Age and Position on Peak Expiratory Flow Rate: A Longitudinal Study. *Obstet. Gynecol.* 2005;105:372-5.

[18] Murphy, V. E., Clifton, V. L., Gibson, P. G. Asthma exacerbation during pregnancy: incidence and association with adverse pregnancy outcome. *Thorax* 2006;61:169-76.

[19] Lao, T. T., Huengsburg, M. Labour and delivery in mothers with asthma. *Eur. J. Obstet. Gynecol. Reprod. Biol.* 1990;35:183-90.

[20] Schatz, M., Dombrowski, M. P., Wise, R., Thom, E. A., Landon, M., Mabie, W., Newman, R. B., Hauth, J. C., Lindheimer, M., Caritis, S. N., Leveno, K. J., Meis, P., Miodovnik, M., Wapner, R. J., Paul, R. H., Varner, M. W., O'Sullivan, M. J., Thurnau, G. R., Conway, D., McNellis, D. Asthma morbidity during pregnancy can be predicted by severity classification. *J. Allergy Clin. Immunol.* 2003;112:283-8.

[21] Schatz, M., Harden, K., Forsythe, A., Chilingar, L., Hoffman, C., Sperling, W., Zeiger, R. S. The course of asthma during pregnancy, post

partum and with successive pregnancies: a prospective analysis. *J. Allergy Clin. Immunol.* 1988;81:509-17.

[22] Murphy, V. E., Gibson, P. G., Talbot, P. I., Clifton, V. L. Severe asthma exacerbations during pregnancy. *Obstet. Gynecol.* 2005;106:1046-54.

[23] Stenius-Aarniala, B., Piirilä, P., Teramo, K. Asthma and pregnancy: a prospective study of 198 pregnancies. *Thorax* 1988;43:12-8.

[24] Gluck, J. C., Gluck, P. A. The effect of pregnancy on the course of asthma. *Immunol. Allergy Clin. North Am.* 2006;26:63-80.

[25] Jana, N., Vasishta, K., Saha, S. C., Khunnu, B. Effect of bronchial asthma on the course of pregnancy, labour and perinatal outcome. *J. Obstet. Gynaecol.* 1995;21:227-32.

[26] Beecroft, N., Cochrane, G. M., Milburn, H. J. Effect of sex of fetus on asthma during pregnancy: blind prospective study. *BMJ.* 1998;317:856-7.

[27] Dodds, L., Armson, B. A., Alexander, S. Use of asthma drugs is less among women pregnant with boys rather than girls. *BMJ.* 1999;318:1011.

[28] Kwon, H. L., Belanger, K., Holford, T. R., Bracken, M. B. Effect of fetal sex on airway lability in pregnant women with asthma. *Am. J. Epidemiol.* 2006;163:217-21.

[29] Bakhireva, L. N., Schatz, M., Jones, K. L., Tucker, C. M., Slymen, D. J., Klonoff-Cohen, H. S., Gresham, L., Johnson, D., Chambers, C. D.; OTIS Collaborative Research Group. Fetal sex and maternal asthma control in pregnancy. *J. Asthma.* 2008;45:403-7.

[30] Firoozi, F., Ducharme, F. M., Lemière, C., Beauchesne, M. F., Perreault, S., Forget, A., Blais, L. Effect of fetal gender on maternal asthma exacerbations in pregnant asthmatic women. *Respir. Med* 2009;103(1):144-51. Epub. 2008 Aug. 29.

[31] Kircher, S., Schatz, M., Long, L. Variables affecting asthma course during pregnancy. *Ann. Allergy Asthma Immunol.* 2002;89:463-6.

[32] Baibergenova, A., Thabane, L., Akhtar-Danesh, N., Levine, M., Gafni, A. Is fetal gender associated with emergency department visits for asthma during pregnancy? *J. Asthma.* 2006;43:293-9.

[33] Enriquez, R., Griffin, M. R., Carroll, K. N., Wu, P., Cooper, W. O., Ebretsadik, .T, Dupont, W. D., Mitchel, E. F., Hartert, T. V. Effect of maternal asthma and asthma control on pregnancy and perinatal outcomes. *J. Allergy Clin. Immunol.* 2007;120:625-30.

[34] Tata, L. J., Lewis, S. A., McKeever, T. M., Smith, C. J., Doyle, P., Smeeth, L., West, J., Hubbard, R. B. A Comprehensive Analysis of

Adverse Obstetric and Pediatric Complications in Women with Asthma. *Am. J. Respir. Crit. Care Med.* 2007;175:991-7.

[35] Källén, B., Rydhstroem, H., Aberg, A. Asthma during pregnancy-a population based study. *Eur. J. Epidemiol.* 2000;16:167-71.

[36] Blais, L., Forget, A. Asthma exacerbations during the first trimester of pregnancy and the risk of congenital malformations among asthmatic women. *J. Allergy Clin. Immunol.* 2008;121:1379-84.

[37] Getahun, D., Ananth, C. V., Peltier, M. R., Smulian, J. C., Vintzileos, A. M. Acute and chronic respiratory diseases in pregnancy: Associations with placental abruption. *Am. J. Obstet. Gynecol.* 2006;195:1180-4.

[38] Perlow, J. H., Montgomery, D., Morgan, M. A., Towers, C. V., Porto, M. Severity of asthma and perinatal outcome. *Am. J. Obstet. Gynecol.* 1992;167:963-7.

[39] Lehrer, S., Stone, J., Lapinski, R., Lockwood, C. J., Schachter, B. S., Berkowitz, R., Berkowitz, G. S. Association between pregnancy-induced hypertension and asthma during pregnancy. *Am. J. Obstet. Gynecol.* 1993;168:1463-6.

[40] Demissie, K., Breckenridge, M. B., Rhoads, G. G. Infant and maternal outcomes in the pregnancies of asthmatic women. *Am. J. Respir. Crit. Care Med.* 1998;158:1091-5.

[41] Liu, S., Wen, S. W., Demissie, K., Marcoux, S., Kramer, M. S. Maternal asthma and pregnancy outcomes: a retrospective cohort study. *Am. J. Obstet. Gynecol.* 2001;184:90-6.

[42] Wen, S. W., Demissie, K., Liu, S. Adverse outcomes in pregnancies of asthmatic women: results from a Canadian population. *Ann. Epidemiol.* 2001;11:7-12.

[43] Norjavaara, E., de Verdier, M. G. Normal pregnancy outcomes in a population-based study including 2,968 pregnant women exposed to budesonide. *J. Allergy Clin. Immunol.* 2003; 111:736-42.

[44] Katz, O., Mazor, M., Wiznitzer, A., Sheiner, E. *Seasonality in Deliveries of Asthmatic Patients.* Presented at the World Asthma Meeting WAM, 22-25 June 2007, Istanbul, Turkey.

[45] Tata, L. J., Lewis, S. A., McKeever, T. M., Smith, C. J., Doyle, P., Smeeth, L., Gibson, J. E., Hubbard, R. B. Effect of maternal asthma, exacerbations and asthma medication use on congenital malformations in offspring: A UK population-based study. *Thorax* 2008;63(11):981-7. Epub. 2008 Aug. 4.

[46] Bracken, M. B., Triche, E. W., Belanger, K., Saftlas, A., Beckett, W. S., Leaderer, B. P. Asthma symptoms, severity, and drug therapy: a

prospective study of effects on 2205 pregnancies. *Obstet. Gynecol.* 2003;102:739-52.

[47] Triche, E. W., Saftlas, A. F., Belanger, K., Leaderer, B. P., Bracken, M. B. Association of asthma diagnosis, severity, symptoms, and treatment with risk of preeclampsia. *Obstet. Gynecol.* 2004;104:585-93.

[48] Dombrowski, M. P., Schatz, M., Wise, R., Momirova, V., Landon, M., Mabie, W., Newman, R. B., McNellis, D., Hauth, J. C., Lindheimer, M., Caritis, S. N., Levenko, K. J., Meis, P., Miodovnik, M., Wapner, R. J., Paul, R. H., Varner, M. W., O'Sullivan, M. J., Thurnau, G. R., Conway, D. L.; National Institute of Child Health and Human Development Maternal-Fetal Medicine Units Network and the National Heart, Lung, and Blood Institute. Asthma during pregnancy. *Obstet. Gynecol.* 2004;103:5-12.

[49] Stenius-Aarniala, B. S., Hedman, J., Teramo, K. A. Acute asthma during pregnancy. *Thorax* 1996;51:411-4.

[50] Bakhireva, L. N., Schatz, M., Jones, K. L., Chambers, C. D.; Organization of Teratology Information Specialists Collaborative Research Group. Asthma control during pregnancy and the risk of preterm delivery or impaired fetal growth. *Ann. Allergy Asthma Immunol.* 2008;101:137-43.

[51] Doucette, J. T., Bracken, M. B. Possible role of asthma in the risk of preterm labor and delivery. *J. Obstet. Gynaecol.* 1995;21:227-32.

[52] Minerbi-Codish, I., Fraser, D., Avnun, L., Glezerman, M., Heimer, D. Influence of asthma in pregnancy on labor and the newborn. *Int. J. Gynaecol. Obstet.* 2002;77:117-21.

[53] Mihrshahi, S., Belousova, E., Marks, G. B., Peat, J. K.; Childhood Asthma Prevention Team. Pregnancy and birth outcomes in families with asthma. *J. Asthma.* 2003;40:181-7.

[54] Sobande, A. A., Archibong, E. I., Akinola, S. E. Pregnancy outcome in asthmatic patients from high altitudes. *Int. J. Gynaecol. Obstet.* 2002;77:117-21.

[55] Linton, A., Peterson, M. R. Effect of preexisting chronic disease on primary cesarean delivery rates by race for births in US military hospitals, 1999-2002. *Birth* 2004; 31:165-75.

[56] Belanger, K., Hellenbrand, M. E., Holford, T. R., Bracken, M. Effect of pregnancy on maternal asthma symptoms and medication use. *Obstet. Gynecol.* 2010;115:559-67.

[57] Wendel, P. J., Ramin, S. M., Barnett-Hamm, C., Rowe, T. F., Cunningham, F. G. Asthma treatment in pregnancy: a randomized controlled study. *Am. J. Obstet. Gynecol.* 1996; 175:150-4.

[58] Källén, B., Rydhstroem, H., Aberg, A. Congenital malformations after the use of inhaled budesonide in early pregnancy. *Obstet. Gynecol.* 1999; 93:392-5.

[59] Schatz, M., Dombrowski, M. P., Wise, R., Momirova, V., Landon, M., Mabie, W., Newman, R. B., Hauth, J. C., Lindheimer, M., Caritis, S. N., Leveno, K. J., Meis, P., Miodovnik, M., Wapner, R. J., Paul, R. H., Varner, M. W., O'Sullivan, M. J., Thurnau, G. R., Conway, D. L.; Material-Fetal Medicine Units Network, The National Institute of Child Health and Development; The National Heart, Lung and Blood Institute. The relationship of asthma medication use to perinatal outcomes. *J. Allergy Clin. Immunol.* 2004;113:1040-5.

[60] Dombrowski, M. P., Schatz, M., Wise, R., Thom, E. A., Landon, M., Mabie, W., Newman, R. B., McNellis, D., Hauth, J. C., Lindheimer, M., Caritis, S. N., Leveno, K. J., Meis, P., Miodovnik, M., Wapner, R. J., Varner, M. W., O'Sullivan, M. J., Conway, D. L.; National Institute of Child Health and Human Development Maternal-Fetal Medicine Units Network; National Heart, Lung, and Blood Institute. Randomized trial of inhaled beclomethasone dipropionate versus theophylline for moderate asthma during pregnancy. *Am. J. Obstet. Gynecol.* 2004;190:737-44.

[61] Rahimi, R., Nikfar, S., Abdollahi, M. Meta-analysis finds use of inhaled corticosteroids during pregnancy safe: a systematic meta-analysis review. *Hum. Exp. Toxicol.* 2006; 25:447-52.

[62] Silverman, M., Sheffer, A., Diaz, P. V., Lindmark, B., Radner, F., Broddene, M., de Verdier, M. G., Pedersen, S., Pauwels, R. A.; START Investigators Group. Outcome of pregnancy in a randomized controlled study of patients with asthma exposed to budesonide. *Ann. Allergy Asthma Immunol.* 2005;95:566-70.

[63] Breton, M. C., Beauchesne, M. F., Lemière, C., Rey, É., Forget, A., Blais, L. Risk of perinatal mortality associated with inhaled corticosteroid use for the treatment of asthma during pregnancy. *J. Allergy Clin. Immunol.* 2010;126:772-777.

[64] Martel, M. J., Rey, E., Beauchesne, M. F., Perreault, S., Forget, A., Maghni, K., Lefebvre, G., Blais, L. Use of short-acting beta2-agonists during pregnancy and the risk of pregnancy-induced hypertension. *J. Allergy Clin. Immunol.* 2007;119:576-82.

[65] Morfín Maciel, B. M., Castillo Morfín, B. M. Theophylline, a new look to an old drug. *Rev. Alerg. Mex.* 2010;57:112-22.

[66] Källén, B., Otterblad Olausson, P. Use of anti-asthmatic drugs during pregnancy. 1. Maternal characteristics, pregnancy and delivery complications. *Eur. J. Clin. Pharmacol.* 2007;63:363-73.

[67] Källén, B., Otterblad Olausson, P. Use of anti-asthmatic drugs during pregnancy. 2. Infant characteristics excluding congenital malformations. *Eur. J. Clin. Pharmacol.* 2007;63:375-81.

[68] Källén, B., Otterblad Olausson, P. Use of anti-asthmatic drugs during pregnancy. 3. Congenital malformations in the infants. *Eur. J. Clin. Pharmacol.* 2007;63:383-8.

Index

B

C

D

E

I

T

U

V

W

Y

Z